Restoration of Motor Function in the Stroke Patient

Restoration of Motor Function in the Stroke Patient

A PHYSIOTHERAPIST'S APPROACH

Margaret Johnstone M.C.S.P.

Illustrated by
Estrid Barton

Foreword by
Professor Bernard Isaacs M.D. F.R.C.P.
Charles Hayward Professor of Geriatric Medicine,
University of Birmingham

CHURCHILL LIVINGSTONE
EDINBURGH LONDON AND NEW YORK 1978

CHURCHILL LIVINGSTONE
Medical Division of Longman Group Limited

Distributed in the United States of America by
Churchill Livingstone Inc., 19 West 44th Street,
New York, N.Y. 10036 and by associated compan-
ies throughout the world.

First published 1978
  Reprinted 1980

ISBN 0 443 01701 8

British Library Cataloguing in Publication Data

Johnstone, Margaret
    Restoration of motor function in the stroke patient.
    1. Cerebrovascular disease   2. Physical therapy
    I. Title
    616.8'1   RC388.5   77-30517

Printed in Hong Kong by
Wilture Enterprises (International) Ltd.

This book is dedicated to Dr David Seaton,
Consultant Physician of Chalmers Hospital,
Edinburgh, who first suggested to me that I should 'let
the stroke patient stand on his hands' and then
encouraged me to put this principle into practice along
with the 'Dott principles' I already used.

Foreword

Margaret Johnstone has already placed her view on stroke rehabilitation before the physiotherapy and nursing professions in her book *The Stroke Patient: Principles of Rehabilitation.* Her justification for returning to the subject is a desire to place in the hands of practising physiotherapists a more detailed account of the progressive steps which she believes to be essential if the fullest potential for recovery of the stroke patient is to be realised. This, she believes passionately, will be achieved if, and only if the physiotherapist adheres throughout treatment to a clear policy firmly based on a profound understanding of the basic neurophysiological principles of recovery in the central nervous system. No physiotherapist, she believes, can afford to be empirical or haphazard in her method of working; no one can take tantalising short cuts to the restoration of function by methods which later break their promise; and leave the patient with an uneasy adaptation to a persistent handicap, rather than a soundly based recovery. How this is to be achieved is set out in a text that brims with the enthusiasm and glows with the devotion of its author. The text is illustrated by drawings of great clarity which leave the reader in no doubt about the precise details of treatment.

In recent years physiotherapy has been undergoing a rapid and exciting movement from an empirical form of treatment to a scientifically based profession. Stroke rehabilitation has lagged in this process. Margaret Johnstone's sincere and compassionate book is a clarion cry to physiotherapists to apply their neurophysiological knowledge to the management of stroke patients; and she holds out, as a reward to her colleagues, the possibility of achieving a high standard of response in this needy group of patients.

Birmingham, 1977   Bernard Isaacs

Preface

The need to present this book as a follow up to my previous book, *The Stroke Patient: Principles of Rehabilitation* has become increasingly obvious to me. It has been written in response to the many questions and appeals for help that I have received from my professional colleagues. I have devoted the last twelve years of my professional life to the consideration of residual stroke problems and, at the same time, I have been deeply involved in the observation, handling and care of stroke victims. This book is an attempt to share with my colleagues the knowledge and understanding I have gained from that experience and, in particular, from the teaching of three outstanding tutors: Professor Norman Dott, Miss M.I.V. Mann and Miss M.D. Gardiner. It offers a way of treatment founded on long experience and sound principles in order to encourage others who find themselves caring for stroke victims to become deeply involved.

For many years the physician has tended to hand over the physical care of his patients to the 'expert' care of the physiotherapist. In some cases, this has been a misplaced trust. In ignorance, some physiotherapists may have offered rehabilitation which has simply built up, or reinforced, the growing patterns of spasticity in the patient's affected limbs. In other cases where there has been gross sensory loss with the resultant useless, heavy, flaccid limb, nothing has been offered towards re-education of this lost sensory function and any chance of rehabilitation has remained quite hopeless.

Speaking in particular to members of my profession, and to be fair to the physiotherapist, it should be said that in many instances the doctor has not been fully aware of the problems facing his stroke patients or of the principles of rehabilitation which must be thoroughly understood if these patients are to be offered a reasonable hope of functional recovery. Frequently, the doctor has taken it for granted that the physiotherapist, as the expert in this field, knows all the answers and will therefore give the patient the fullest possible chance of a return to normal living. If we think about this, we must realise that we would not have it otherwise. As physiotherapists we ought to be experts. Rehabilitation is our subject and if we have not always offered expert treatment, we should ask ourselves, 'Where have we gone wrong?'.

A recent and encouraging sign that many of us acknowledge our shortcomings but are not prepared to accept them is seen in the large numbers of our profession who queue up to attend lecture courses in order that we may bring understanding to bear on the difficulties encountered in this very specialised field of rehabilitation. We have begun to ask the question; 'Are we good enough?'. If we reach the conclusion that physiotherapy has not done well enough, and that the numbers in the recovery group who go back to a useful life have not increased, we must then conclude that we are *not* good enough. There must still be gaps in our knowledge and flaws in our treatment. Worse still, in some cases by offering the bad handling that comes with lack of understanding of the problems involved, we may sometimes have actively prevented the recovery that might otherwise have taken place.

It is possible that the Romans were ahead of us in the treatment of their stroke victims. Hot baths where passive movements and active assisted movements were given in the water was the order of the day, and it is reasonable to suppose that this treatment was followed by skilled massage and exercises which included rolling over to prone. Our record of successful treatment in modern times has not been spectacular, the high percentage of failure with these patients has led many of us to despair and we are left with the uncomfortable feeling that we ought to be able to do better.

But we must not look back. We must go forward. We must accept full responsibility. The physiotherapist must be the expert, she must be prepared to lead the rehabilitation team and, where necessary she must be prepared to demonstrate the correct method of positioning and of handling these patients so that they are given every chance of recovery and of reaching out with *both* hands to grasp at an independent future. To do this, she herself must have a thorough understanding of the problems her patient has to face, she must understand the basic principles of this specialised rehabilitation, and she must strive to reach a point where she can join with her professional colleagues to say with every confidence; 'We *are* good enough'. We will only reach this point when we know that we are offering rehabilitation treatment of a very high standard to all stroke victims and that we substantially increase the numbers in the recovery group who go back to a useful life.

It will be understood then, that this book is a professional testimony addressed by one physiotherapist to her professional colleagues and it sets out a personal method of treatment. I think it would be fair to say that my treatment has been broadly based on what I now find to be a reasonable understanding and interpretation of the Bobath concept. The Bobath principles are comparatively new to my experience; I had not studied Bobath until fairly recently, but I had used what I choose to refer to as the Dott principles. I was fortunate enough to be taught by Professor Norman Dott and to work for him in his wartime unit for gunshot wounds of the head. I spent many years developing my stroke treatments round principles based on the firm foundation he gave me. Added to this, I have developed a new method of treatment which depends on deep pressure to inhibit dominant reflexes and to step up sensory input while, at the same time, making early weight-bearing from the heel of the hand through an extended elbow to an externally rotated shoulder possible from a very early date after onset of the stroke. It gives the stability of sustained posture that is necessary for successful rehabilitation.

The techniques suggested in this book do not offer a short-cut to a successful outcome, they simply offer a treatment routine that will give the stroke patient a reasonable hope of returning to normal living. The process of integrating reflex mechanisms involved in controlled movement will, of necessity, take time and I see no reason to change the already accepted attitude where recovery time is considered in months rather than in weeks. Sensory development and motor development progress together and cannot be separated. This means that both are involved in all stages of treatment; both are involved where rolling techniques are used to lead towards the ability to adopt and hold a sitting position; both are involved where postural and righting reflexes are called into action by alterations of the head in space and in relation to the trunk and extremities.

Throughout the text there is of necessity a repetition of basic principles. This has been found to be necessary because successful stroke rehabilitation depends on building slowly with tedious and persistent repetition on exercise routines which ought not to move forward beyond the individual patient's capability and which must be founded, at every stage, on sound principles. I have found over the years that the average physiotherapist who is looking for help in establishing these routines asks to have these basic principles repeated with every progression made in an advancing treatment programme.

There are some who will feel that the section on assessment ought to have been placed at the beginning of the book. In answer to this criticism I would suggest that the ability to make an accurate assessment depends on full understanding of the problems that may be encountered, plus a certain expertise that only comes with experience. How to handle the stroke patient has therefore been fully discussed first. It must always be remembered that an early, hasty assessment will tend to be unreliable. At the end of four weeks after the onset of a stroke the average patient is able to perform the initial bed exercises, will roll freely from side to side, prop and balance on the affected elbow and sit in a chair with good sitting balance if he has been handled correctly from the beginning. At the end of four weeks the average patient is ready to have a reliable assessment made. But, again, it must be remembered, the performance may vary from day to day.

It may be said that I make extravagant claims for the use of pressure splints in stroke treatment. I would not agree. My findings are based on a ten year trial period during which time I have had consistently good results. Given the already established facts that it is necessary to inhibit dominant reflexes to prevent developing spasm (that is, by using careful positioning at all times), and that it is also frequently necessary to step up sensory input, I would suggest that the pressure splint fulfils both of these necessities *if* it is applied with the limb in the inhibited position and *if* it is inflated sufficiently to give deep, all-over, even pressure. I would also suggest that any success I may claim is a direct result of developing a method which simultaneously inhibits dominant reflexes while facilitating sensory impulses to make rehabilitation possible. I find that the pressure splint has given me the missing link—or the perfect aid—in the sensorimotor approach I make to stroke rehabilitation, re-establishing the finely balanced facilitory-inhibiting principle on which the neuromuscular system depends.

In records I have kept while using the method presented in this book, none of the patients treated has developed the all too common painful shoulder that, in the past, effectively prevented the rolling and weight-bearing progressions necessary for successful rehabilitation and I have come to expect return of arm function. I would suggest that if any of my professional colleagues are tempted to challenge my assumption that consistently good treatment results must serve as suitable evidence to present my case for the use of pressure splints without running independent clinical trials, they might pause to consider the neurophysiological principles behind my assumptions and they might also consider that no other effective method of dealing with the residual problem of the hemiplegic arm has yet been offered. With the pressure splint re-establishing the finely balanced facilitory-inhibiting principle on which the neuromuscular system depends it is then possible by repetition and graduated and increasing demand to re-establish purposeful movement. As far as I am concerned, clinical trials would mean withholding the treatment that has proved itself by a high rate of success over a lengthy period from 50 per cent of my patients and condemning them to my former treatments where the success rate was low and the residual problems indissoluble. Added to this, as no two strokes are exactly the same, results would be inconclusive.

The nearest approach to a control study that I have made is to compare and contrast my treatment results with the poor rate of success I obtained prior to my use of pressure splints. I have also recently spent two years working in a long stay unit where it was possible to find many examples of the neglected stroke case of long standing. With the aid of pressure splints I found it was possible to relieve the distress caused by the tightly fisted hand and the resulting comfort given made late treatment well worthwhile. But in the text of this book I have not set out to discuss late treatment, I have rather presented the case for the early, intensive and repetitive treatment that leads to success in the non-progressive lesion.

It is not the purpose of this book to go deeply into the anatomy of the nervous system and the notes I offer on neurology are brief and consequently incomplete. For example, believing that the physiotherapist must understand the need to plan a rehabilitation programme which depends for its success on making use of anti-gravity mechanisms and tonic postural reflexes, the factors which maintain normal muscle tone have been touched on very briefly. But control of muscle tone is far more complex than suggested here, in particular the cerebellum, reticular formation and basal ganglia play extremely important roles. In attempting to simplify the very complex mechanisms of muscle tone, postural control and proprioception, inaccuracies may have crept in. It is impossible to be wholly brief and wholly accurate. Considerable extension of the scope of this book would be necessary if neurology were to be covered thoroughly from every aspect. As the book has been conceived specifically to help physiotherapists in the restoration of motor function in the stroke patient, it has been presented solely as a rehabilitation manual and not as a comprehensive medical textbook. In my experience, few, if any, fully understand the whole complex working of the human brain—certainly not the average physiotherapist—and those who are deeply involved in caring for stroke patients will already have made a careful study of the nervous system. Suggestions for further reading are included at the end of the book.

The attitude of the physiotherapist to her work and to her patient is of first importance. No physiotherapist can afford to forget that, in part, her success rate in this highly specialised type of rehabilitation depends on her ability to pass on to her patient a belief in recovery and a return to home living. Where there is no prospect, or no belief in the prospect of a return to home life, rehabilitation is usually slow and limited. So I make no excuse for offering a second book on stroke rehabilitation; it is devoted entirely to physical re-education and should be of interest to anyone who handles stroke patients, to all the staff of a well-integrated rehabilitation team, but in particular it is addressed to the physiotherapist. We must move forward together in understanding and we must interpret our understanding into sound principles of rehabilitation. I am confident that we need not despair, there is a hopeful future for all stroke patients with a non-progressive lesion, and there is no valid reason for us not to be equal to facing this challenge.

In conclusion, I would like to thank Professor Isaacs for the understanding and the help he has given me. Without his encouragement I would not have set out to write this book and I am very grateful for his support. I also owe a great deal to the publishers, particularly to Miss Mary Emmerson for her invaluable advice and help. They have strengthened my belief in my work and helped me to put this book together so that it may fill a gap in the literature that has already been published on this specialised and fascinating field of rehabilitation.

Edinburgh, 1977   M.J.

Acknowledgements

Professor Isaacs of the University of Birmingham who encouraged me to write this book.

Dr Walsh, medical director of Parke-Davis, who kept me supplied with pressure splints when they were difficult to obtain so that I might continue my research into the residual problem of the hemiplegic arm.

Miss Estrid Barton, who spent a summer vacation sketching me at work in my stroke unit and so making it possible to write the script round her drawings.

Mrs Victoria Hards, Superintendent Physiotherapist of Liberton Hospital, Edinburgh, whose understanding and help has been invaluable.

Miss R. Lane and her very special rehabilitation team who confirmed and strengthened my belief in my approach to stroke rehabilitation in a recent visit I made to Aberdeen.

Dr John Scott, Consultant Geriatrician, Woodend General Hospital, Aberdeen, who assisted me in my first book *The Stroke Patient: Principles of Rehabilitation* and gave me every encouragement to go ahead with this one.

Mrs Ann Thorp, my sister and fellow physiotherapist, who has encouraged and assisted me in our recent venture into the field of lecture demonstrations.

Dr H.M. McLeod, Consultant Geriatrician, Liberton Hospital, Edinburgh, for the interest he has taken in my work and for his invaluable assistance in seeing that I was supplied during the last two years with the apparatus I needed to continue working in the difficult area of sensory loss.

Contents

1. Controlled Movement

In the beginning

This book should be of interest to all who have dealings with stroke patients and, in particular, to those who are actively engaged in handling stroke patients. It is written from the point of view of rehabilitating the patient who has a non-progressive lesion. Therefore, it does not offer any quick method which would of necessity take short-cuts. It does not give suggestions for gaining some degree of independence as soon as possible without any regard for the final outcome. To do that would be to teach the patient to compensate with his sound side. When we set out to rehabilitate patients with a non-progressive lesion, we must recognise that these are the patients who ought to be considered to be in the full recovery group. They must be given the chance of returning to a normal life. In other words, treatment must rehabilitate the missing function and establish the full independence of a whole body. No patient who rehabilitates by learning to compensate with his sound side ever returns to normal living.

Throughout the text of this book, in order to avoid confusion, it is assumed that the patient is male and the physiotherapist is female.

To make a start, it is necessary to go right back to the beginning and remember exactly what happens to the patient who has a stroke, leaving other disabilities that might be present (apraxias, dysphasia, agnosias and so on) until a later chapter and beginning with the immediate physical disability.

The missing function that faces all stroke patients:
    1. Loss of the normal postural reflex mechanism on the affected side and, therefore, inability to initiate movement on this side.
    2. Developing hypertonicity (spasticity) in the anti-gravity muscles.
    3. Usually some degree of sensory disturbance which inhibits movement.
    4. Consequently there is a complete loss of free selection of precision movements on the affected side.
    It is the job of the physiotherapist to help her patient to keep developing spasm at a minimum while she teaches him how to regain his lost function. To do this she must have a thorough understanding of the problems he faces.

1

The postural reflex mechanism

In order to make a realistic and efficient approach towards stroke rehabilitation it is first necessary to fully understand what is meant by:
1. Skeletal muscle tone
2. Reflex action
3. Labyrinthine reflexes
4. The postural reflex mechanism.

This will lead to a clear understanding of the true nature of the physical disability that has overtaken the stroke patient.

1. *Skeletal muscle tone*

During all our waking hours our voluntary muscles, even when they are at rest, are always maintained in a state of mild contraction and this is called tone. Muscle tone is present to some extent in all voluntary muscles but it is more marked in the muscles which hold the body upright against gravity—mainly the extensors of the lower limbs, trunk and neck. In the upper limbs, the forearm flexors may be classed as anti-gravity muscles because they are used to lift and to carry weight against gravity. In the ape, along with the shoulder depressors, the forearm flexors are used to lift the body weight against gravity. Thus the extensors of the lower limbs, trunk and neck and the forearm flexors and shoulder depressors all belong to the group of muscles in which skeletal muscle tone is more marked than elsewhere. Muscle tone is entirely reflex in character and is maintained by reflexes which produce changes in tone in relation to noxious stimuli and weight transference. A lesion of the corticospinal tracts gives exaggerated tonic contraction—complete separation of the lower centres from higher control giving an extreme degree of increased muscle tone.

2. *Reflex action*

A reflex action is an involuntary action resulting from stimulation of a sensory nerve ending, e.g. the quick recovery of balance (or centre of gravity) if the toe is caught on the edge of the pavement. In any reflex action a large number of reflexes are involved. Place a hand on a very hot surface and this immediately activates the muscles of the arm, shoulder, trunk, neck, tongue, voice, larynx, eyes and respiration to name the obvious muscles which are at once involved in the resulting reflex action (or withdrawal response). The number of motor neurones involved in this reflex action is far greater than the number of sensory endings which stimulated it, so the sensory (or receptor) neurone must be connected with a large number of motor (or effector) neurones. This is a valuable asset in our rehabilitation programme for our stroke patient.

Receptor, or sensory, endings can be either exteroceptors (receiving stimuli from the external environment), proprioceptors (receiving stimuli from within the body itself), or interoceptors (receiving stimuli from air and food) which are found in the mucous membrane of the respiratory and alimentary tracts. Of these, the proprioceptors play the most important part in stroke treatment.

3. *Labyrinthine reflexes*

It must be remembered that the ear is not simply the organ of hearing. The inner ear, or labyrinth, as well as containing the receptors of hearing also contains the three semicircular canals and two small sacks, the utricle and the saccule. These semicircular canals and the utricle have nothing to do with hearing, their function is solely concerned with the maintenance of equilibrium. The semicircular canals and the utricle respond to movement in different ways—the canals respond to movements of the head in space whereas the position of the head acts on the hair cells of the utricles; that is, the first responds to movement, the second to position. This is the phenomenon that gives us the *labyrinthine righting reflex* which produces changes in extensor tone with changes in the position of the labyrinth, a mid-brain response. Thus, when the head is moved in space it triggers off a reflex mechanism—or stimulates the labyrinthine righting reflex—which is best illustrated by following the actions of, for example, a dog when he is placed on his back, or wrong way up. He will immediately right himself. He turns his head to move it into its accustomed position in space, his body follows his head, the sequence of muscle action being contraction of neck muscles followed by contraction of trunk and limb muscles. To follow the reflex action right through, remember that neck movements stimulate proprioceptors in the neck muscles (neck reflexes being an upper cervical response) and this in turn initiates reflex righting movements of the trunk and limbs. So, by reflex action, a mid-brain response and an upper cervical response have been stimulated, labyrinthine righting reflex leading to stimulation of neck proprioceptors, and it must be remembered that these reflex actions are involuntary.

4. *The postural reflex mechanism* (N.B. closely concerned with the vestibular system, see Glossary)

This mechanism consists of three main factors, normal postural tone and its adjustment, normal reciprocal innervation and normal patterns of coordination. This is the mechanism which we do not have when we are born. It develops in the infant stages of kicking, rolling, crawling, kneeling and standing, or along the parallel lines of rolling to sitting to standing and rolling to prone lying to propping to crawling to standing. The postural reflex mechanism develops from tonic reflex levels and labyrinthine reflexes as described above—*spinal* and *tonic* levels leading to *basal* level where righting reflexes and equilibrium responses are developed. Righting reflexes and equilibrium responses include a cortical element and, as soon as they are thoroughly established, *cortical* level (with voluntary responses and learned skills) takes over (see Fig. 1). Note that all levels from *spinal* upwards can be modified but **basal**

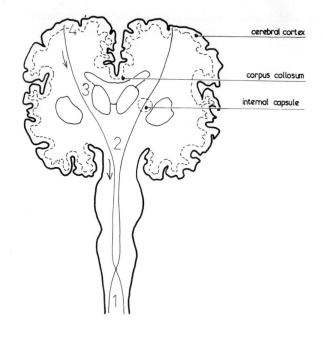

1 = SPINAL   Spinal reflex level

2 = TONIC   Mid-brain responses / Tonic neck reflexes / Labyrinthine reflexes

3 = BASAL   Righting reflexes / Equilibrium responses

4 = CORTICAL   Voluntary responses

NOTE : All levels from 1 upwards can be modified <u>BUT</u>
       3 is required before 4 can be effective.

FIG.1: DIAGRAM OF THE BRAIN TO SHOW LEVELS OF REFLEX ACTIVITY.

response is necessary before **cortical** *response can be effective.* This fact gives one of the main points which must be understood and used as a guide line when working out the rehabilitation programme of each stroke patient.

Note: It should be helpful to study Figure 1 and to read and become thoroughly familiar with the following notes. If the development of the postural reflex mechanism is not understood it will be impossible to make a reasoned and realistic approach to stroke rehabilitation.

As the study of the development of the *postural reflex mechanism*

becomes familiar we recognise the different levels of reflex activity as:
1. *spinal*
2. *tonic*
3. *basal*
4. *cortical*

We can follow the development of this reflex mechanism quite simply if we follow through these four stages.

1. *Spinal:* giving tonic reflexes.

Tonic reflexes are reflexes which produce involuntary changes in muscle tone in response to stimulation of sensory nerve endings— exteroceptors and proprioceptors. Of these we are most concerned with stimulation of the proprioceptors in response to changes of the body's position in space (e.g. by rolling) giving pressure on soft tissues and weight transference.

There are three distinct types of tonic reflex. (i) The positive supporting response: which gives an increase in extensor tone in a limb bearing weight. (ii) The negative supporting response: which gives a decrease in extensor tone when weight is taken off a limb. (iii) The withdrawal response: (as described above) which gives an increase in flexor tone in response to undesirable stimulation.

These are involuntary reflex happenings but must be understood if re-education of the postural reflex is to be undertaken.

2. *Tonic:* giving tonic labyrinthine reflex and tonic neck reflexes.

These are stereotyped primitive responses which are modified or overruled at higher levels when the postural reflex mechanism is fully established. They play a very important role in stroke rehabilitation.

(i) The tonic labyrinthine reflex obviously depends on an intact spinal cord and brain stem. The receptor organs are the labyrinthine canals of the inner ear as described above. As the afferent pathway influences the vestibular nuclei, causing these neurones to send excitatory impulses to fusimotor fibres of extensor muscles and so increasing reaction to stretch stimuli, this reflex increases extensor tone. Because of this reflex, the position of the head has a fundamental bearing on muscle tone.

(ii) The tonic neck reflexes relate to the position of the cervical spine and, again, the afferent pathways influence the vestibular nuclei, but the pattern of increased muscle tone differs in relation to any altering position of the cervical spine. Two quite distinct patterns may be demonstrated.

(a) The symmetrical tonic neck reflex results from *flexion* or *extension* of the cervical spine. With flexion, extensor tone increases in the lower limbs and decreases in the upper limbs. With extension, extensor tone decreases in the lower limbs and increases in the upper limbs.

(b) The asymmetrical tonic neck reflex is related to *rotation* of the cervical spine. For example, if the head is turned to the left there is an increase in extensor tone in the limbs of the left side and a decrease in extensor tone in the limbs of the right side—or vice versa.

3. *Basal:* giving righting reflexes and equilibrium responses.

A combination of righting reflexes makes up a righting response while equilibrium responses are very complex mechanisms which develop from righting responses. They can only be touched on in the simplest of terms and in a very simple manner in a book of this length.

(i) The head righting reaction follows movement of the head in space with correction of eye level in response to disturbance of the labyrinth. The head rights, movement of the cervical spine stretches the neck muscles and triggers off the reflex mechanism to bring the body into alignment of head, neck and trunk. This leads to controlled rolling, controlled rolling to sitting, and finally to the ability to rotate within the body axis and, therefore, to controlled movement, rotation being a necessary component of normal movement.

(ii) Equilibrium responses follow in the development pattern. Tonic reflexes, which give changes in muscle tone with weight transference, combine with righting responses to give automatic shifts in tone all over the body which relate to position changes, making possible the patterns of movement necessary for daily living. These are the responses which are required to carry out any action smoothly against gravity, to 'place' a limb and to 'hold' at rest, to 'hold' against gravity and to maintain balance. Equilibrium responses, therefore, include shifts in muscle tone with compensating movements to allow the body to stand up to any altering situation caused by changes of position or environment. When fully developed, equilibrium responses allow us to support our weight over a fixed base, or, if necessary, to find a new base. They allow us to 'prop' over a fixed base and to maintain this fixed base while reaching out in any direction, to maintain balance against an external opposing force, or to regain lost balance by reaching out, hopping or side-stepping.

4. *Cortical:* giving voluntary responses and learned skills.

It is important to note that all levels from 1 to 4 can be modified but **righting reflexes and equilibrium responses must be established before cortical level can be effective.** This means that to attempt to take a short cut in stroke rehabilitation, neglecting to establish righting reflexes and equilibrium responses, will leave a missing link in the recovery chain and ruin the patient's chances of returning to a normal life.

The anti-gravity mechanism of the human body, and in particular the reflexes mentioned above which are so closely concerned with obtaining an upright position and correct body alignment, must be used in stroke rehabilitation if rehabilitation is to be effective. Wherever there is a regression of motor skills to a more primitive level with loss of controlled movement, of equilibrium responses, possible perceptual difficulty and loss of sensory discrimination, it is necessary to go back to the beginning and start rebuilding on a firm foundation. It makes sound sense to think of the reflex arc as the basic functional unit of the nervous system and to seriously consider a course of rehabilitation which builds on this basic unit. It may be helpful to include brief notes on the *functional areas of the cerebral cortex.* For purposes of easy description each cerebral hemisphere is divided into four lobes—frontal, parietal, occipital and temporal (Fig. 2).

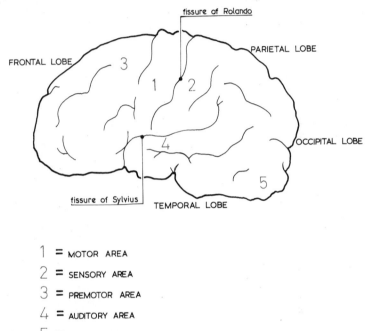

1 = MOTOR AREA
2 = SENSORY AREA
3 = PREMOTOR AREA
4 = AUDITORY AREA
5 = VISUAL AREA

FIG.2: DIAGRAM OF FUNCTIONAL AREAS IN THE CEREBRAL CORTEX.

The frontal lobe contains the motor area responsible for voluntary movement. This area may be subdivided into foot, ankle, knee, hip, trunk, shoulder, elbow, wrist, hand, neck, face, tongue and larynx—working from above downwards. These areas connect with the motor cranial nuclei and the anterior horn cells, crossing to the opposite side of the body in the corticospinal tracts.

The parietal lobe contains the sensory area. Kinesthetic sense is perceived and interpreted in this area, the body parts being in the same order from above downwards as in the motor area. Kinesthetic sense results from the impulses set up by the stimulation of proprioceptors in muscles, tendons and joints though all do not reach consciousness but end in the central nervous system. Where there is parietal lobe involvement in the stroke patient, rehabilitation may present tremendous problems and may need many months of careful treatment if effective response is to be gained.

The occipital lobe contains the visual area. It is important to remember that impulses from the left halves of the retinas are transmitted to the visual area of the left hemisphere, impulses from the right halves of the retinas to the right hemisphere. This means that where there is destruction of the visual cortex on the right side of the brain there will be hemianopia involving the right halves of both retinas. The adjacent area of the occipital lobe is concerned with recognition of visual impressions and their interpretation and integration with other sensations. Those caring for stroke victims must be able to distinguish between hemianopia and visual agnosia. These problems will be dealt with much later in the text.

The temporal lobe contains the acoustic area, or the centre for hearing, each centre receiving impulses from both ears. Thus destruction of one centre produces some dullness of hearing but not total deafness. The area immediately adjacent to the centre for hearing is responsible for interpretation of sound and, therefore, with understanding the meaning of sounds and the associations of sounds with other sensations.

No serious attempt to cover the anatomy of the nervous system is made here, but in these brief notes which are simply offered as an aid to the understanding of stroke care, there is one other structure of the brain that probably ought to be mentioned. This is the internal capsule.

The internal capsule is the name given to a structure composed of bundles of ascending and descending nerve fibres—the corticospinal and sensory tracts concern us most. The internal capsule separates the basal ganglia from the thalamus and it is the narrow pathway for all motor and sensory fibres going from the cortex to lower levels, and for all sensory fibres ascending from lower levels to the cortex. Damage to the conducting pathways leads to loss of power in the muscles on the side of the body opposite to the site of the lesion.

Thus the characteristic feature of the stroke patient is loss of willed movement of one side of the body and this is accompanied by an upset of postural tone. Postural tone may be increased, or decreased, or both. Where it is increased it is described as spasticity, or hypertonicity, and where it is decreased as flaccidity, or hypotonicity. Stroke, or hemiplegia, most usually results from cerebral thrombosis or haemorrhage and more usually starts with an initial flaccid stage which moves on to a residual spastic stage. This state of spasticity is a result of increased muscle tone due to release of abnormal reflex activity. In other words, the dominant reflexes are no longer inhibited from the higher centres of the brain because of damaged pathways. Stroke, when it occurs in the young adult, is more likely to be the result of a cerebral embolism caused

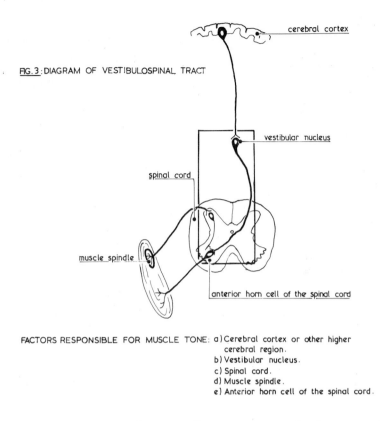

FIG.3 : DIAGRAM OF VESTIBULOSPINAL TRACT

cerebral cortex

vestibular nucleus

spinal cord

muscle spindle

anterior horn cell of the spinal cord

FACTORS RESPONSIBLE FOR MUSCLE TONE: a) Cerebral cortex or other higher cerebral region.
b) Vestibular nucleus.
c) Spinal cord.
d) Muscle spindle.
e) Anterior horn cell of the spinal cord.

by rheumatic or bacterial heart disease, or the result of rupture of a congenital aneurysm, or of an angioma.

The vestibulospinal tract (see Fig. 3). Muscle tone and its maintenance by the spinal reflex arc has been considered. Also, when considering labyrinthine and tonic neck reflexes it has been stated that extensor tone is reinforced by impulses from the vestibular nuclei. *The vestibular nuclei are inhibited by higher centres. If isolated from these higher centres, hyperactivity results* which gives excessive tone—or spasticity. This means that the higher centres must be effective to achieve the final desired balance of normal muscle tone. Remembering that righting reflexes and equilibrium responses must be established before cortical level can be effective, the vestibulospinal tract is considered here in order to emphasise the need for *early rehabilitation. The main aim of treatment is to rehabilitate normal patterns of movement.* The essential requirement necessary to make this aim possible is to prevent the development of the abnormal patterns of movement which result from abnormal tone. If allowed to develop, these movements effectively put an end to all worthwhile rehabilitation. To prevent this from happening it is essential to begin treatment immediately after the onset of the stroke and, throughout the whole treatment programme, to use methods which *inhibit dominant reflexes,* or, in other words, to use methods which *hold developing spasm at a minimum.*

Conclusion: All true stroke rehabilitation begins at spinal level and works upward. Where rehabilitation is carried out with understanding of the levels of reflex activity and the need to build on the reflex arc—the basic functional unit of the nervous system—treatment should go forward with little or no difficulty to the mutual enjoyment and satisfaction of the patient and the physiotherapist *provided it is possible to inhibit dominant reflexes* at all times. All levels of reflex activity have been touched on but the structural basis of reflex action, the reflex arc, has not been discussed, nor has it been suggested how dominant reflexes might be brought under control until muscle tone has been restored.

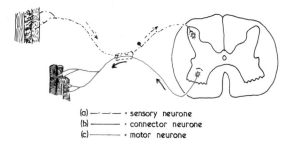

(a) — · — · — · sensory neurone
(b) ——————— · connector neurone
(c) ——————— · motor neurone

FIG. 4 : DIAGRAM OF SIMPLE REFLEX ARC.

The reflex arc (Fig. 4), the basic functional unit of the nervous system, is illustrated here in its simplest form showing a receptor neurone, a connector neurone and an effector neurone. Stimulation of the sensory nerve ending gains a response from the motor neurone. This is a monosynaptic arc and, in man, it is only found in the phasic stretch reflexes of muscles, e.g. the knee jerk response elicited by tapping quadriceps tendon. Most reflexes are polysynaptic where the afferent supply enters the central nervous system at the segmental level dictated by the receptor organ and the motor response occurs at many levels because connecting interneurones transmit impulses to countless motoneurone pools at *lower and higher levels.* A more detailed account of reflex mechanisms makes a fascinating study but it is beyond the scope of this book to go more deeply into the background of reflex activity behind the development of skilled movement. Suffice it to point out that response to afferent stimulation gains a response at many levels.

The whole rehabilitation programme is based on redevelopment of controlled movement in response to reflex activity. For this reason I have discussed the development of the postural reflex mechanism in comparative detail. But another illustration ought to be given. It will be helpful to consider this development from the outside rather than from the inside.

Development of controlled movement in the baby

Motor development in the baby is from head to foot in direction, that is proximal to distal, or neck and shoulder before arm and hand, trunk and hip before leg and foot. Foetal movements are reflex movements and are called primitive, but it must be remembered that these primitive reflex movements are the predecessors of all purposeful, coordinated actions. At birth, the first movements are still primitive—eye movements, head turning, kicking, finger grasp and so on. Most of us have watched these restless, primitive movements of the newborn child, and later, as the baby grows and the development of motor function continues we have seen these primitive movements develop into controlled movement which can be performed deliberately or automatically. We have been watching the baby develop his postural reflex mechanism. He learns to roll. Rolling is a new movement. He repeats it again and again as if he is practising his new trick—as, indeed, he is. With the constant repetition of this new movement, and because of the alterations of the position of his head in space and in relation to his trunk and extremities, postural and righting reflexes are called into action. Soon rolling from supine to prone becomes a controlled and functional movement and he rolls to prop on his forearms or he rolls into sitting, the more complicated equilibrium responses developing. He extends his head in prone and he crawls on his forearms dragging his legs. Forearm crawling leads to pushing himself backward and he gets onto all fours. Supporting himself in this position he pushes himself backwards and forwards over his hands, freeing his primitive flexor grip and releasing his hands for functional movement. Postural stability and controlled movements progress; he pulls himself up on to his feet, he bears weight, shifts his weight, transfers it from foot to foot, develops postural stability, the primitive movements of flexion and extension are modified and he walks.

This fascinating sequence of motor development can be followed in any healthy infant moving from birth through the beginning months of life. It is the outward and visible sign of inward and invisible reflex action, controlled movement and postural stability developing concurrently with the development of the nervous system. From intensive repetition of primitive movements which gain a reflex response he has developed controlled movement.

In the stroke victim we are faced by half of a whole human being. With his postural reflex mechanism cut off from cortical control, he is unable to initiate movement from his affected side and he is therefore not in full command of his neuromuscular system. Unless we re-educate the missing function, re-establishing cortical control, he will never again be

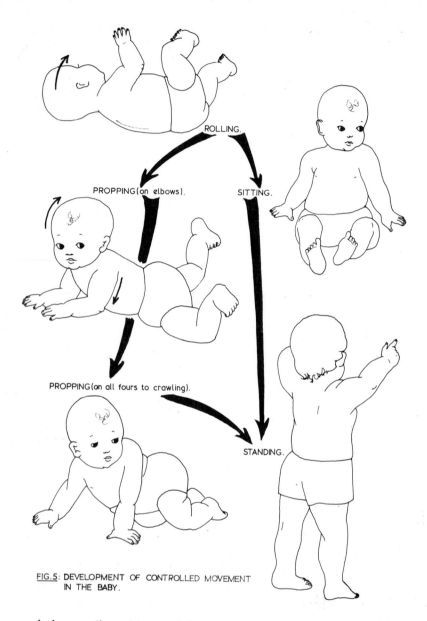

ROLLING.

PROPPING(on elbows).

SITTING.

PROPPING(on all fours to crawling).

STANDING.

FIG.5: DEVELOPMENT OF CONTROLLED MOVEMENT
IN THE BABY.

a whole, coordinated human being capable of initiating movement from either, or both, sides of his body and capable of living a normal and free life.

This means, that within the limit of fatigue, the stroke patient must learn to roll and he must repeat the exercise over and over again, as did the baby, the aim being to promote optimum recovery of righting reflexes and equilibrium responses—which are in part cortical responses so as to lead back to cortical control and therefore to rehabilitate selective, coordinated, purposeful movement.

It is helpful to stress the sequence of movement used in early rehabilitation exercise. Eyes move first followed by the head followed by movement of the body. The physiotherapist's voice directed at the patient from his affected side is used to stimulate his *hearing* and his *vision*. His eyes move in response and his head follows, *hearing* and *vision* giving the initial *sensory stimulation*. (Wherever necessary, hearing aids must be checked to make sure that they are in full working order). Sensory feed-back has a very important part to play in all successful rehabilitation and the physiotherapist must be included as part of this necessary feed-back. We have been taught that sensory development and motor development move forward together in the infant and so with our stroke patient they are inseparable; re-education of the one must assist re-education of the other.

Gross movements, or primary trunk movements, return first, followed by movements from proximal to distal—that is, shoulder to elbow to hand, or hip to knee to foot. As the baby develops it becomes obvious that the arms are ready to be used in controlled movement before the legs are ready for full weight bearing and controlled walking patterns. This should not be surprising as we realise that rolling to elbow propping comes earlier than propping on all fours, or kneeling, in the baby's programme of development, and standing on the hands comes before standing on the feet (see Fig. 5). This propping ability plays a large part in the development of postural responses and therefore it should play a major part in our rehabilitation programme.

The sequence of development is from proximal to distal—shoulder to elbow to hand—but the test of full recovery of controlled selective movement is the final rehabilitation of the distal to proximal sequence—hand to elbow to shoulder. This most important final step in re-education cannot be obtained unless the patient has been taught to follow, step by step, the stages of motor development as seen in the normal programme of motor development in the human baby. Remembering that the purpose of this book is to present a considered and worthwhile approach to the *complete* stroke due to a non-progressive lesion, where other factors, e.g. the patient's age, make mat routines difficult a way round the extra disability must be found. Should the stroke be due to a progressive lesion, the approach would be entirely different. In this case the patient would probably be taught to compensate with his sound side in an attempt to speed up his return to what must then be an expected limited period of semi-ambulant, one-sided living.

It will by now be understood that any course of treatment which sets out to rehabilitate controlled movement in the stroke patient will encounter a disturbance of postural tone which will present special problems which must be recognised and which must be tackled if success is to be the outcome.

Conclusions so far reached:

1. With dysfunction of the postural reflex mechanism and where dominant reflexes are no longer under cortical control—or the vestibular nuclei are no longer inhibited at higher level—spasticity will develop. Therefore, treatment aims at re-establishing the normal postural reflex mechanism.

2. In the developmental approach to treatment suggested here, weight must be borne on *upper* and lower limbs to stimulate underlying postural reactions, e.g. the positive supporting reflex, and to fully integrate righting and equilibrium reactions and must include pressure to the sole of the foot and the *palmar surface of the hand.*

3. No conclusion has so far been reached about the problem presented by developing spasticity.

2. Positioning

The problem of developing spasticity

The previous section considered muscle tone and its maintenance by the spinal reflex reinforced by impulses from the vestibular nuclei. With the vestibular nuclei isolated from higher centres, the resulting hyperactivity leads to hypertonus of muscles—or spasticity. In all effective rehabilitation of the stroke patient it is essential to re-establish the normal postural reflex mechanism, which includes cortical control, but this cannot be done *unless developing spasticity is held at a minimum* while rehabilitation is undertaken.

In other words, with the stroke patient, cortical control is lost; the static postural reflexes are no longer under cortical control and are no longer integrated into functional movement patterns. The result is abnormal tonic reflex activity giving the typical picture of the spastic hemiplegia.

Spasticity develops in the anti-gravity muscles and there is no difficulty in deciding which are the anti-gravity muscles if the activities of an ape are considered. He uses his legs to stand upright against gravity making leg extensors into anti-gravity muscles, and he *externally* rotates his hips. He uses shoulder depressors with *internal* rotation and forearm flexion to pull his body weight up into a tree against gravity. This illustration gives a graphic picture of the anti-gravity muscles which are involved and should lead to a clear understanding of the *spasm pattern* that will develop in the stroke patient if no preventive measures are taken. This may be considered by some to be a rather outdated analogy but I include it because it serves very well to illustrate the stronger muscle groups and the synergic pattern of tonic contraction will shortly follow as a result of uninhibited dominant reflexes. One other fact must be taken into account. Latissimus dorsi belongs to the strong group of depressor muscles of the shoulder and the action of latissimus dorsi is to draw the shoulder downwards and backwards into retraction with *internal* rotation. (The opposite pattern is protraction with elevation and *external* rotation). Because of the size and origins of this very large muscle it is reasonable to suppose that there will be lateral trunk shortening on the stroke patient's affected side.

The pattern of spasticity in the stroke patient bears a direct relationship to the dominating reflexes and these are the reflexes which are

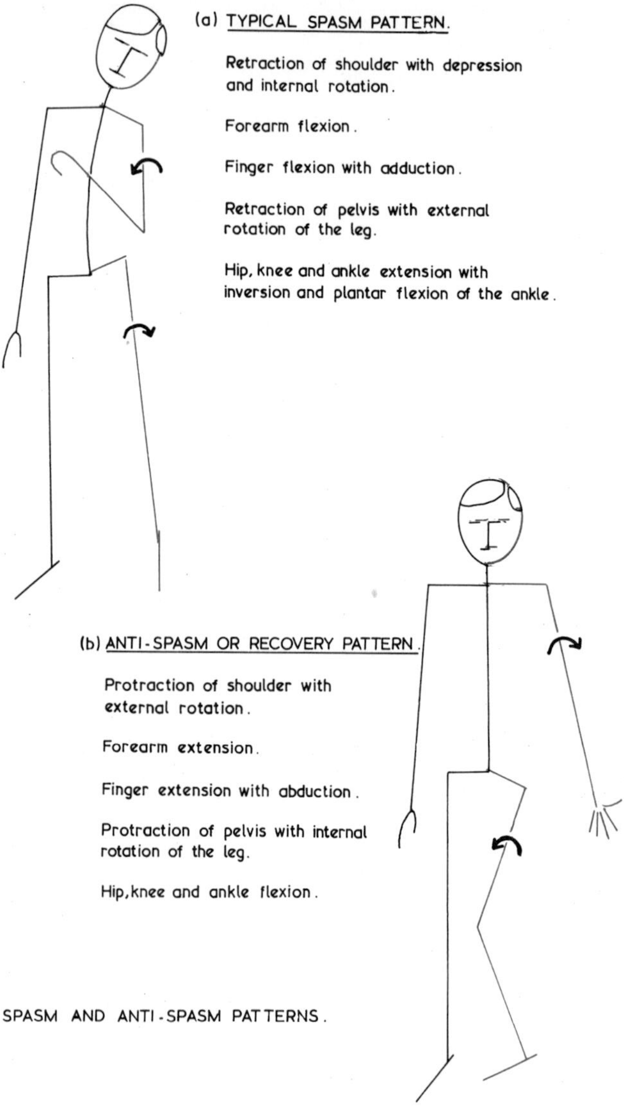

(a) TYPICAL SPASM PATTERN.

Retraction of shoulder with depression and internal rotation.

Forearm flexion.

Finger flexion with adduction.

Retraction of pelvis with external rotation of the leg.

Hip, knee and ankle extension with inversion and plantar flexion of the ankle.

(b) ANTI-SPASM OR RECOVERY PATTERN.

Protraction of shoulder with external rotation.

Forearm extension.

Finger extension with abduction.

Protraction of pelvis with internal rotation of the leg.

Hip, knee and ankle flexion.

FIG.6 : SPASM AND ANTI-SPASM PATTERNS.

modified at cortical level when the postural reflex mechanism is fully established.

Using the illustration of an ape pulling himself by his arms to hoist himself into a tree, or extending his legs to push himself upright against gravity, it is a simple matter to work out the typical pattern of spasticity that can be expected to develop in the stroke patient. Figure 6a gives a diagrammatic representation of this pattern.

Typical spasm pattern

As might be expected, there is:

(a) Retraction of the affected shoulder with depression and *internal* rotation.

(b) Forearm flexion, usually accompanied by pronation.

(c) Finger flexion with adduction.

(d) Retraction of the pelvis with *external* rotation of the leg.

(e) Hip, knee and ankle extension with inversion and plantar flexion of the ankle.

(f) Lateral flexion of the trunk to the affected side.

This is the pattern of spasm that can be expected to develop very quickly after the onset of a stroke. In the typical stroke patient spasticity follows the usual brief initial flaccid stage and develops over a period of a year to eighteen months, and this is the situation that challenges all of us who set out to rehabilitate stroke patients. It should be possible to re-educate missing function by early, intensive and repetitive treatment involving rolling, prone lying, elbow propping, kneeling, crawling ... and so on, moving up through the levels of reflex activity, *but* while this programme is carried out it is a sad fact that developing spasticity usually outstrips rehabilitation and effectively puts an end to all worthwhile treatment.

It is not surprising that the following statements seem to contradict each other: (1) While rehabilitation is carried out developing spasticity must be held at a minimum. (2) As long as there is lack of cortical control, spasticity will develop. It looks like a vicious circle with no way out. But there is a way out. The answer lies in positioning. *Positioning* consists of using the anti-spasm (or recovery) pattern at all times. From the day of onset the patient must be placed in the anti-spasm pattern and all exercise must lead into recovery patterns. If the typical spasm pattern (Fig. 6a) has been understood, understanding of the anti-spasm pattern ought not to present any difficulty. It is quite simply the pattern which is in direct opposition to the spasm pattern and is shown in Fig. 6b.

The anti-spasm pattern

(a) Protraction of the shoulder with *external* rotation.

(b) Forearm extension with supination.

(c) Finger extension with abduction.

(d) Protraction of the pelvis with *internal* rotation of the leg.

(e) Hip, knee and ankle flexion.

(f) Elongation of the trunk on the affected side.

So it will be seen that the spasm pattern in the stroke patient, as in all neurological conditions, involves total patterns of movement and, therefore, *if allowed to develop,* it will prevent re-education of all normal patterns of voluntary movement on the affected side. Because of the loss of normal inhibiting influences on motor neurones from cortical level, the reflex activity of muscles which act as antagonists against gravity is no longer controlled and the resulting hyperactivity gives the typical spasm pattern as described above. There is too much motor unit activity because there is too little inhibition of motor neurones from cortical level. In the stroke patient we talk about the *synergic pattern of tonic contraction* which results from hypertonic, or excessive, muscle tone in the anti-gravity muscles (as described above) giving muscle contraction which follows the pattern of the synergists. In other words, the fine balance between reciprocal relaxation and co-contraction is thrown out of gear and the synergists (which contract and relax in conjunction with the prime movers *crossing more than one joint*) upset normal coordination by excessive co-contraction. This demonstrates in the stroke patient as developing spasticity which is accompanied (because of the synergic pattern) by loss of *rotation*. It is this developing spasticity with loss of rotation that must be held in check by diligent positioning of the patient at all times. The general weakness which accompanies the spasticity on the affected side, as will be expected, is most severe in the flexors of the leg and the extensors and elevators of the arm.

If the reference to anti-gravity muscles in the ape confuses some who will maintain that we no longer swing from trees by our arms, it may be useful to remember that anti-gravity for the human arm means forearm carrying muscles flexing against gravity and reinforced by the strong action of latissimus dorsi giving shoulder depression with internal rotation. It must also be remembered that in the normal child, where the fully established reflex mechanism has led to full development of controlled movement, cortical level is fully established and controlled movement includes voluntary responses and learned skills. To re-educate the stroke patient to his former ability, which must include cortical control, it will now be understood that it is necessary to prevent developing spasticity during the entire rehabilitation programme.

It has been said that in stroke rehabilitation, where there is sensory loss, the physiotherapist must be included as part of the sensory feed-back. It is important to stress here that she must also act as *the inhibiting influence on hypertonic motor neurones* until the missing postural reflex mechanism is re-established and normal inhibiting influences restored. She acts as this inhibiting influence by making sure that she— and all her team—maintain the stroke patient in the anti-spasm pattern twenty-four hours a day. In other words, correct positioning is used as an inhibiting influence on hyperactive motor neurones (or developing spasm) until inhibition from cortical level is re-established.

It is not enough to understand the anti-spasm or recovery pattern. It is also necessary to gain experience in handling stroke patients and to work with them until it becomes second nature to handle them correctly, to position them correctly, and to use every daily activity (from, for example, the initial use of a bed-pan) as an exercise in the rehabilitation of lost motor control. If we are dealing with a patient who has a non-progressive lesion, lost motor function will be regained if every activity is accompanied by diligent positioning.

To gain some understanding of the full meaning of diligent positioning, consider the use of the affected hand in rehabilitation. Referring to Figure 6b, the anti-spasm pattern for the arm gives external rotation of the shoulder with forearm extension and finger extension with abduction. In terms of the hand, this means extension of the wrist with

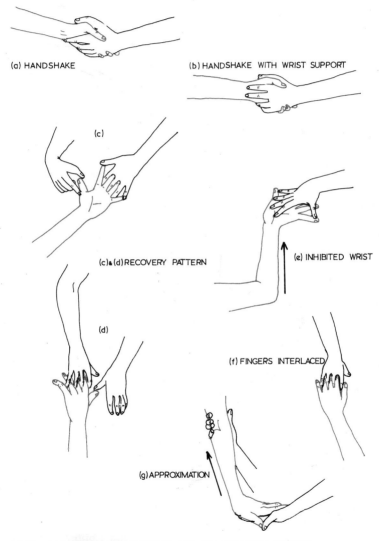

(a) HANDSHAKE

(b) HANDSHAKE WITH WRIST SUPPORT

(c)

(c)&(d)RECOVERY PATTERN

(e) INHIBITED WRIST

(d)

(f) FINGERS INTERLACED

(g) APPROXIMATION

FIG.7(a-g): HANDGRIPS USED TO WORK INTO THE RECOVERY PATTERN.

external rotation (supination) and extension with abduction of all fingers and the thumb. This means that at all times, all or some part of this anti-spasm pattern should be in use. Now consult Figure 7. This shows handgrips used to work into the anti-spasm (or recovery) pattern, maintaining correct positioning while rehabilitation is in progress. The red hands represent the patient's affected hand, the black hands are those of the physiotherapist, the nurse, or any member of the rehabilitation team. A brief description of each handgrip will serve to show what is meant by using, or working into, the anti-spasm pattern.

Handgrips used to work into the recovery pattern

(a) *The handshake grasp:* is used frequently in the early stages of handling the stroke patient. With the patient in lying, sitting or standing, this handgrip may be used to keep the thumb uppermost, turning the hand away from pronation and into supination and keeping the shoulder in external rotation.

(b) *Handshake with wrist support:* is a variation of the simple handshake. The extra wrist support which is given by the physiotherapist's first and second fingers gives useful wrist control.

(c and d) *The recovery pattern:* holds the fingers in the full recovery pattern and is used in many of the arm rehabilitation exercises.

(e) *Recovery pattern with inhibited wrist:* repeats the full recovery pattern of the hand and full wrist extension is added as an additional inhibiting influence. The elbow is placed in flexion and weight is supported from elbow to hand (approximation). It will later be seen that for hand recovery it is essential to use this position in rehabilitation and it ought to be used as early as possible in the treatment programme before wrist extension is lost.

(f) *Fingers interlaced:* holds the patient's fingers in the required abduction position. This position also gives the physiotherapist a useful grip for passive and active assisted exercise making sure that external rotation is maintained at the shoulder. It also leaves the physiotherapist with a free hand to hold the affected shoulder well forward in protraction.

(g) *Approximation:* this time from hand to shoulder (or shoulder to hand), the wrist is extended and the thumb abducted. Again, this leaves the physiotherapist with a free hand to stabilise the elbow in extension. It will be shown that correct handling of the stroke patient is almost always approached from the affected side by *one* person and this handgrip will be used repeatedly.

These handgrips, properly used, all keep well within the anti-spasm pattern. Elbow flexion must obviously be used quite frequently in the rehabilitation programme, but, where it is used, care is taken not to allow the shoulder to turn inwards to the forbidden spasm pattern of internal rotation. In the diagram (Fig. 7e) it is shown in use with the wrist inhibited and the shoulder in external rotation. Following through the rehabilitation programme, the use of these handgrips will become thoroughly familiar—or second nature—and this gives a fair illustration of what is meant by using and working into the anti-spasm (or recovery) pattern at all times.

In the same way, positioning of the body as a whole must be understood and, as far as possible, must be maintained at all times. As soon as it is understood, correct positioning will be used at all times as a matter of course. It is quite usual to find that where it is used as a rigid routine, the patient very quickly begins to position himself or to ask for help towards maintenance of correct positioning. Adequate supporting pillows must be available. To assist all those who are setting out to become efficient and experienced workers in the stroke rehabilitation team a series of diagrams is included which shows very clearly the anti-spasm pattern in practice. Figures 8 to 24 show the positions which must be established and used early in the rehabilitation programme. Figures 8 to 10 give the resting positions which ought to be used at all times of resting, and which must be maintained by adequate supporting pillows while the patient is resting in bed.

The artist's model was a young healthy male who was prepared to hold the required positions for lengthy drawing sessions and, in some instances, adequate supporting pillows were not used because they would have interrupted the clear view of the correct position. The drawings are self-explanatory but a brief commentary to pinpoint and enlarge on the important details is included below.

All the initial diagrams in the book on the correct positioning and handling of the stroke patient ought to be understood and carefully followed by all members of the stroke rehabilitation team and, in particular, this must include nurses as well as physiotherapists.

Correct positioning and early handling of the stroke patient

Lying on the back: or supine (Fig. 8), is the position which must be used with the greatest care because it is the position which produces maximal extensor spasticity, giving retraction or a dropping backwards of the arm into internal rotation and full extension of hip and knee with external rotation of the leg—the complete spasm pattern. Therefore, when supine lying cannot be avoided the greatest care is necessary to position the patient in the anti-spasm pattern. The affected shoulder must be lifted forward (or protracted) and held in this position by a suitably placed pillow with the shoulder in external rotation, elbow and wrist extended. Similarly a pillow is placed under the hip to prevent retraction or a dropping backwards of the pelvis with external rotation of the leg—again the spasm pattern. The pillow holds the hip in protraction and the knee is flexed with internal rotation of the hip. Supporting pillows may be placed under the thigh. Care is taken to elongate the trunk on the affected side and the head is placed in lateral flexion towards the sound side. Where the patient can tolerate the position the neck ought not to be flexed by supporting pillows. In the diagram (Fig. 8), protraction and external rotation of the shoulder is well illustrated and, in order to make these two points suitably clear, the required elevation of the arm is not so clearly shown. The required leg position is exaggerated in order to stress the necessity for knee flexion with protraction, flexion and internal rotation of the hip.

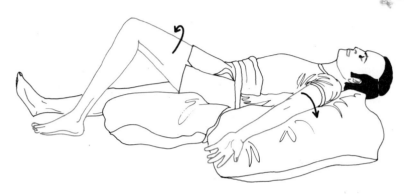

FIG.8: LYING ON THE BACK.

Lying on the sound side: is a good position provided the patient is in full side lying making it easy to place the affected limbs in the anti-spasm pattern. Again the affected shoulder must be protracted, or brought forward, and this is achieved quite simply by placing the affected arm well forward across a supporting pillow with the elbow and wrist extended. Thus the arm cannot fall into internal rotation. The perfect position is obtained by rotating the shoulder externally so that the palm of the hand faces the head of the bed. The affected leg is placed forward giving good hip protraction with the hip and knee in a natural position of flexion. A supporting pillow may be used for comfort. On the other hand, if a pillow is not placed under the head the trunk will lie in a good position because the resulting flat bed will cut out lateral neck flexion to the affected side and will help to keep the trunk in the required elongated position.

Lying on the affected side is also very suitable provided care is taken to position the affected limbs. Again the affected shoulder must be placed well forward in protraction with the elbow and wrist extended. The hand will be in the supine position (palm uppermost) because the shoulder is in the required external rotation. The affected leg lies in a comfortable position with slight flexion of hip and knee. Also for comfort, the sound leg is placed well forward in flexion on a supporting pillow. Note that *when this position is used for exercise* (Fig. 10), the affected leg should be as far as possible in *full hip extension with the knee flexed to 90°* for some part of the exercise session. This is because

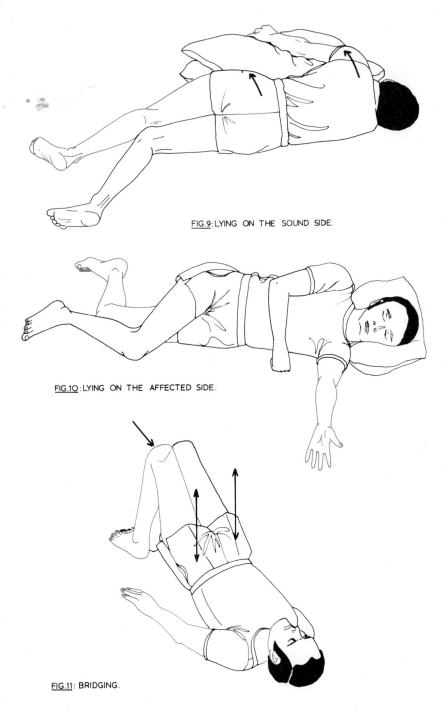

FIG.9: LYING ON THE SOUND SIDE.

FIG.10: LYING ON THE AFFECTED SIDE.

FIG.11: BRIDGING.

full hip extension on the affected side is easily lost. If the maintenance of full hip extension is not taken into account in the early stages of treatment it will later give considerable trouble and will hinder the rehabilitation programme.

Bridging is the fourth position that must be considered in the early days of treatment (Fig. 11) and the correct starting position for bridging ought to be taught at the beginning of the rehabilitation programme. The exercise consists of lying on the back with both knees flexed and lifting the hips up to balance in this position. From a nursing point of view, this is a necessary exercise for the delivery of a bed-pan and it is also useful when the patient can use it freely because it enables him to take his weight off his buttocks at frequent intervals, maintaining comfort and reducing any risk of developing pressure sores. The crook position—lying on the back with knees flexed and held firmly together to prevent outward rotation at the hips—is also the position it is easiest for the patient to maintain to prevent build up of extensor spasm in the affected leg when supine lying cannot be avoided. If the position is to be held for any length of time, correct positioning of pillows will assist shoulder protraction. Symmetrical neck flexion using supporting pillows ought not to be encouraged. Active flexion of the sound leg helps to tilt the pelvis forwards and initiates active holding in flexion of the affected leg. In the beginning it may be necessary for the nurse or physiotherapist to hold the affected leg in the required crook position and assist the pelvic raising. If the patient is large, awkward or confused, he may need the assistance of two people to establish the exercise. The nurse and the physiotherapist ought to be prepared to work together. They should take up their positions, one on either side of the bed. With a single wrist grasp under the small of the patient's back they assist the lifting of his hips while they hold his knees in position. The physiotherapist will stabilise the crook-lying position first, then the bridging position with hips raised. Crook-lying will be stabilised from the knees, bridging from the hips. Active assisted movement into the bridging position will lead to active movement followed by resisted movement which will be given bilaterally and unilaterally. Each progression is introduced as soon as the patient is able to take an active part in the exercise. Bridging *must* be established and performed as an early independent exercise and will be used as an early essential exercise position as well as for nursing purposes. Early weight bearing is a necessary feature of stroke rehabilitation if full recovery is to be obtained and bridging is the first exercise in early weight bearing. Lifting the hips off the bed brings the trunk muscles on the affected side into action, initiating hip movement and assisting in proximal recovery—in other words, assisting in re-establishing controlled and functional movement of the hip. Bridging also plays an important part in preparation for standing up and sitting down and, later, a mobile pelvis will be an essential part of stable, rhythmical walking. It should also by now be fully understood that this exercise keeps well within the necessary anti-spasm pattern. In my experience, the patient who fails to establish bridging, fails to establish a normal walking pattern.

Correct positioning for *lying on the back, lying on the sound side, lying on the affected side* and *crook-lying* for bridging are all essential features of early nursing of the stroke patient. They are also the basic early rehabilitation positions and must be used correctly if they are to give the sound base on which successful rehabilitation will be built. It is essential that both the nurse and the physiotherapist should understand the reasoning behind this need for diligent positioning at all times. It will also add enormously to the nurse's feeling of job satisfaction if she realises that, by taking meticulous care over the correct positioning of her patient at all times, she will also play a vital role in his recovery of lost function. Indeed, without her understanding and help in this essential establishment of correct positioning in the first days after the onset of the stroke, the patient's chance of joining the recovery group who return to lead a normal life will be greatly reduced—if not destroyed.

By careful positioning the physiotherapist, or the nurse, must act as *the inhibiting influence on hypertonic motor neurones* until the postural reflex mechanism is re-established, or until the static reflexes once more become integrated into controlled movement—which happens when normal inhibiting influences have been restored. In other words, at all times, correct positioning is used to replace the inhibiting influence that is missing from cortical level. As already described, the spasm pattern bears a direct relationship to these dominating reflexes. Therefore, the side-lying positions, which do not facilitate the spasm pattern, are used whenever possible.

If it is remembered that righting reflexes, as already described, lead to head righting—or correction of eye level in response to disturbance of the labyrinths following movement of the head in space—the logical sequence of rehabilitation is easily understood. The head rights, the body follows the head, leading to alignment of head, neck and trunk. This leads to controlled rolling, controlled rolling to sitting, and so on. Thus it is understood that until the rehabilitation programme reaches the stage where the static reflexes which produce extensor spasticity are fully integrated into controlled movement, side-lying and rolling will be used in part to control extensor spasticity. Tonic neck reflexes are stereotyped primitive responses and should always be taken into account in the early days of rehabilitation. The effects of neck flexion, extension and rotation must always be considered and should be used judiciously in positioning and in active exercise.

As soon as the patient is conscious, active assisted and active rolling is begun. Careful positioning must be included. Prior to this, passive rolling will usually take place in general nursing procedure where the patient is unconscious. In this instance, rolling from side to side (or two hourly turning) is essential. If nurses have not been instructed in the correct positioning to be used, this may be because the physiotherapist has failed to establish the team approach necessary for the best care of these patients. The positioning for lying on the sound side and on the affected side is clearly shown in Figures 9 and 10 and these are the positions which the nurse must use when she turns her stroke patients. Therefore, balance in side-lying in these positions is established early. For resting positions an adequate number of supporting pillows must be available. For example, when lying on the sound side (Fig. 9) the affected leg is placed on a supporting pillow; when lying on the affected side (Fig. 10), the sound leg is placed on a supporting pillow and one or two pillows may be placed to give comfortable support to the sound arm. Note that the affected arm must not be trapped under the body with a retracted shoulder. To allow this to happen is to actively prevent rehabilitation and to set in motion the long painful process of the agony shoulder.

Rolling can either be a mass flexion pattern or an extension pattern. As seen in the beginning stages of the early development of controlled movement in the human infant, it is a mass flexion pattern and it is used as such in this early stage of stroke rehabilitation. Later it will be shown how rolling can be modified to include neck extension and so assist in the re-education of the forearm.

Active rolling to the sound side is initially a very difficult exercise. To roll to the sound side the patient is taught to lead with his eyes and his head follows, the sequence of movement being eyes, neck, shoulders, arms, hands, trunk, legs and feet. The nurse or physiotherapist must stand on the patient's sound side and, if necessary, she will step up sensory input in three ways:

1. *Hearing:* By the clear command in her voice:'Roll towards me!'
2. *Vision:* He moves his eyes and turns his head to see her.
3. *Touch:* She lays her hands firmly on his affected shoulder and hip to assist his movement.

To teach the patient to hook his sound foot under his affected leg to assist the turn is to teach him a habit which will ruin the correct sequence of development of controlled movement and later pose very difficult rehabilitation problems. It turns a rather difficult manoeuvre into a relatively simple one if the patient is taught to clasp his hands in front of his body in elevation. The head turns and the sound side assists the affected side with shoulder rotation which is quickly followed by trunk rotation, legs following automatically. The handclasp position with palms touching also prevents the affected arm from falling backwards and inwards into the forbidden spasm pattern while the shoulder is held well forward in protraction. The handclasp position with palms touching will be used frequently in the rehabilitation programme. Not only does it hold the affected fingers and thumb in the required abduction position and prevents the shoulder from turning in to internal rotation, it also helps the patient to be aware of his affected side and to maintain contact with it.

In the very early days after onset of the stroke, the nurse or the physiotherapist may find it necessary to assist the patient's turn to his affected side by placing her hands over his scapula and buttock as shown in Figure 12.

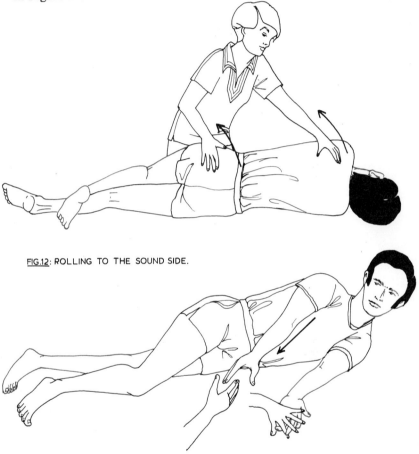

FIG.12: ROLLING TO THE SOUND SIDE.

FIG.13: ROLLING TO THE AFFECTED SIDE.

He will roll with comparative ease on to the affected side but the affected arm must be carefully positioned (Fig. 13). If he maintains the handclasp position to roll to the affected side and carries the arms well forward with protracted shoulders, the arm will automatically finish the movement in the correct position. While balancing in the correct position on the affected side he should be encouraged as soon as possible to reach forward to attempt a more positive and active trunk rotation as shown in Figure 13—gross movements, or primary trunk movements, being the first controlled movement to be re-educated. Very soon he will use this movement to roll and reach across to his locker (which is therefore placed on his affected side) and he will reach across to his locker frequently when he is in bed and so a primary exercise in rehabilitation becomes an exercise in self-care and a useful step towards

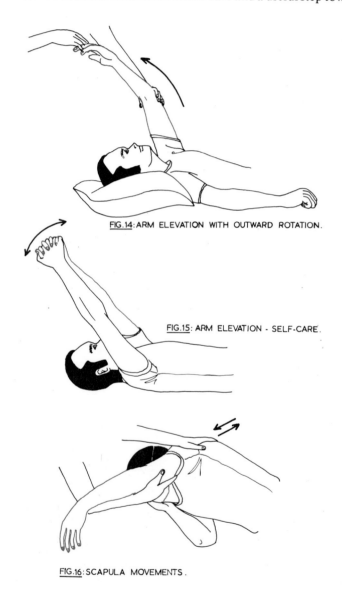

FIG.14: ARM ELEVATION WITH OUTWARD ROTATION.

FIG.15: ARM ELEVATION - SELF-CARE.

FIG.16: SCAPULA MOVEMENTS.

independence. In this simple way the vital exercise of rolling is begun and correctly established in the very early days.

Shoulder and hip care

In the very early days after the onset of a stroke the shoulder and the hip must have special attention if the prospect of the patient's return to a normal life is not to be seriously jeopardised. Once again, the only way of treatment that offers a real prospect of success is to maintain diligent positioning at all times and to work within the anti-spasm pattern. This means the position for these two important joints must be:

Shoulder: protraction with *external* rotation

Hip: protraction with *internal* rotation

It must also be remembered that lying on the back, or supine, is the position which produces maximal extensor spasticity. Shoulder exercise in supine lying must therefore be carried out only after careful positioning of the affected leg in the anti-spasm pattern—hip protracted with *internal* rotation, plus hip, knee and ankle flexion. As soon as crooklying for bridging has been established, the patient will maintain this position with comparative ease and mild rotation of both hips towards the sound side will give the required internal rotation of the affected hip. In the early days supporting pillows will help to maintain and control the essential positioning. In the same way, hip exercise will be carried out only after the affected arm has been carefully positioned in elevation on supporting pillows in the anti-spasm pattern—shoulder protracted with *external* (or outward) rotation, plus forearm extension. A head pillow to give neck flexion for comfort will be used at the discretion of the physiotherapist. Using tonic neck reflexes to increase extensor tone will play an important part at a later stage in rehabilitation of the affected forearm.

Shoulder care in the early days is well illustrated in Figures 14, 15 and 16. While maintaining protraction of the shoulder with external (or outward) rotation, full elevation of the arm must be an early exercise. It will be practised in supine lying as illustrated in Figures 14 and 15—remembering to position the legs as described above. Scapula movements must also be given with the patient lying on his sound side as illustrated in Figure 16.

External rotation of the shoulder with full elevation of the arm is a position which many physiotherapists fail to establish. It is all too easy to start the movement correctly, palm facing upward and thumb pointing away from the body, but as the arm is raised above the head the shoulder is allowed to rotate into the forbidden spasm pattern—internal rotation. If the shoulder is maintained in the required external rotation throughout the exercise, at the end of the movement the thumb will still point away from the body (see Fig. 14) and the palm will still face upward towards the head of the bed. From the point of view of inhibition of spasm and shoulder mobilisation this exercise is of first importance and the correct external rotation of the shoulder joint must be maintained throughout the exercise. In Figure 15, the self-care arm elevation exercise, an acceptable degree of external rotation of the shoulder is maintained by the clasped hands, *palms touching*. The physiotherapist may also assist the patient to practise arm elevation in side-lying (on the sound side) and she may then more easily include extension of the upper spine to use the tonic neck reflex to assist forearm extension.

It is important to note that if early shoulder elevation gives pain the physiotherapist may look for two possible causes.

1. The patient has not been nursed with due care and correct positioning has not been maintained.

2. The arm is not being held in the correct anti-spasm pattern and it is not being moved in the correct groove. It must not be a spiral and diagonal movement.

If correct positioning is maintained from the beginning and correct patterns of movement are established early, shoulder contraction with pain should not occur. Any tendency towards developing spasticity (which demonstrates at first in the fingers) and the resulting contracture (which demonstrates at first in the shoulder) will be prevented or, at worst, will be minimal. The scapula must be kept freely mobile. As stated above therefore, scapula movements should also be given with the patient lying on his sound side. The physiotherapist places one of her hands over the scapula on the affected side and supports the affected arm in external rotation with her other hand and forearm. She is then in a good position to support the affected arm and maintain shoulder protraction while she gives scapula movements in full range (Fig. 16).

Hip care in the early days, as has already been described, begins immediately after the onset of the stroke with careful positioning in mild flexion and internal rotation. As soon as the crook-lying position necessary for bridging has been established it may be said that active hip control has begun. To practise hip rotation in the early days it is usually necessary for the physiotherapist to support the affected leg in the crook-lying position and both knees are then moved as one. A progression is made by using the half-crook-lying position on the affected side with a pillow placed under the affected hip to prevent retraction of the pelvis while internal and external rotation is given. Active internal rotation in particular will be encouraged and the hip must always be returned to the mid-position, retraction with external rotation being part of the spasm pattern. Placing the leg over the edge of the bed and lifting it up again with the knee flexed is necessary so that full range of movement into hip extension is not lost (see Fig. 17). Full hip extension must not be lost or it will later prove very difficult, if not impossible, to establish stable, rhythmical walking. It will be seen from the diagram that this is a passive, or assisted, exercise which, at a later stage when hip control is further developed, will become an active assisted exercise and finally, very much later in the rehabilitation programme, an active movement. Where this programme of hip care (which includes positioning, bridging, rotation, flexion and extension) is carefully undertaken in the early days, a sound beginning towards establishing controlled and functional movement of the hip has been made and proximal recovery has begun.

Knee care in the early days has already been described with careful positioning at all times in mild flexion and in early weight-bearing in bridging. With the leg over the side of the bed as in Figure 17, assisted

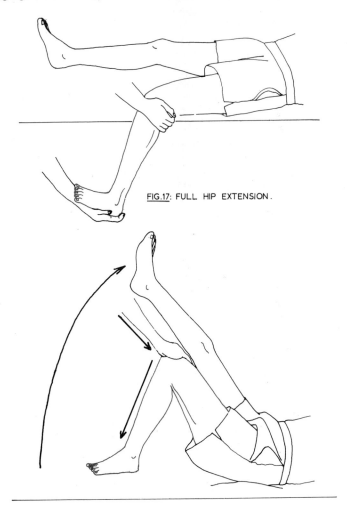

FIG.17: FULL HIP EXTENSION.

FIG.18: EARLY WEIGHT BEARING WITH HAMSTRING CONTRACTION.

knee exercise in mid-range will also be given. Figure 18 shows an effective exercise which will initiate contraction of the hamstrings. Good knee function is frequently thought of in terms of good quadriceps control but hamstring control is equally important and, in stroke rehabilitation, it is particularly important.

An important footnote: Sitting up in bed

It may be necessary to sit the patient up in bed before he is allowed to get out of bed. Again, positioning is all important. In this instance the patient ought to be well up the bed and propped with the help of pillows in an upright position preventing lateral flexion of the trunk to the affected side. Again the affected shoulder is protracted in external rotation with the arm placed well forward on two pillows. The affected leg must not be allowed to roll into external rotation. The first of the supporting arm pillows may be placed on the bed with the edge nearest the patient supporting the lateral side of the affected thigh so that protraction and a mild degree of internal rotation is encouraged in the hip together with mild knee flexion. *A supporting footboard should not be used.* This is because the resulting pressure on the fore part of the foot would reinforce unwanted muscle tone in the leg. It must also be remembered that the positioning of the ward furniture is of primary importance and *the locker must be placed on the patient's affected side.* If we are dealing with a left-sided stroke the locker will be placed on his left hand side. Provided the affected shoulder has been correctly positioned the patient will be taking an active and useful part in his own rehabilitation every time he rotates his shoulders over his pelvis and reaches across his body towards the locker. It must be remembered that rotation of the shoulders over the pelvis (a mass flexion pattern) is an important extensor spasm-inhibiting pattern. Also, by working with the sound side of the body across the midline to the affected side, bilateral activity is initiated by this exercise in *cross facilitation.*

Cross facilitation

Cross facilitation is defined as working with the sound side of the body across the midline to initiate bilateral activity. This technique is widely used in the rehabilitation of the stroke patient; it has been used in rolling in bed, in turning to reach towards the locker, and it will continue to be used throughout the entire rehabilitation programme.

Getting out of bed unaided

In all good stroke rehabilitation, getting out of bed ought to be established as an independent exercise in self-care very early in the treatment programme. Figures 19 to 24 show the stages in progress that ought to be undertaken. Each position ought to be thoroughly established and then incorporated into a progressive treatment plan that will hasten the patient's independence and satisfactory recovery.

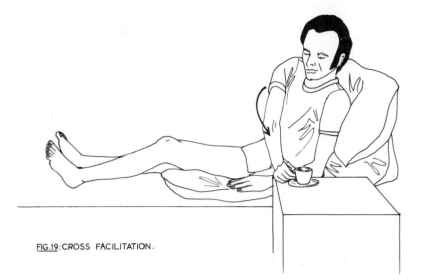

FIG.19: CROSS FACILITATION.

Figure 19 shows propping on the affected elbow in a constructive exercise in cross facilitation as described above. Rolling to prop on the affected elbow must be included in early bed exercise. Remembering spinal tonic reflexes and the positive supporting response, elbow propping will give an increase in extensor tone and, provided the shoulder is correctly positioned, extensor tone must be stimulated repeatedly in the upper limb if recovery is to be obtained. We have already established that early weight-bearing is an essential feature of successful treatment. Here the patient is weight-bearing from elbow to shoulder. The baby turned primitive movement into controlled movement by rolling to propping in his development of motor function.

Figure 20 shows rolling to elbow propping to sitting—or rolling to sitting. This must again be a mass flexion pattern (as in the early development of the baby) and the patient rolls to the affected side. The sequence of movement is rolling to prop on the affected elbow and the sound leg is lifted across the affected leg. It must be noted that the patient is *not* taught to hook his sound leg under his affected leg to lift the affected leg out of bed. This would ruin the whole sequence of the rolling pattern on which the rehabilitation programme is based. (A further small section on the reasoning behind the use of the rolling sequence in stroke rehabilitation will be included at the beginning of the chapter on sensory loss). In rolling to sitting the handshake grasp is used as illustrated in Figure 7a or b. This leaves the physiotherapist or the nurse with a free hand which she cups under the affected heel to assist the movement to sitting. If in any doubt about the assistance given to the

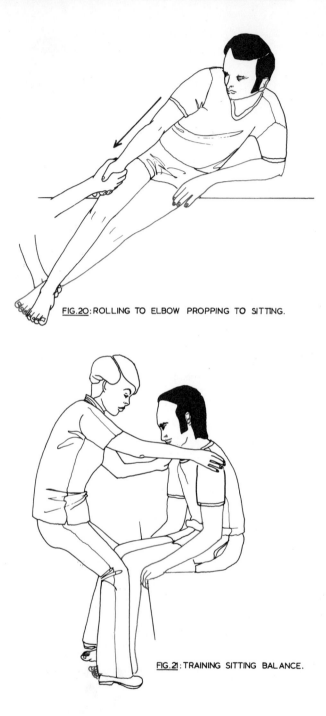

FIG.20: ROLLING TO ELBOW PROPPING TO SITTING.

FIG.21: TRAINING SITTING BALANCE.

patient, study Figure 20. Using this method we are quite clearly following the example set by the infant in motor development, and rolling to sitting with the legs over the edge of the bed very quickly becomes a relatively easy exercise. In a minority of cases rolling to sitting can only be established with the help of two people—but it must be established and in the sequence described above. In the majority of cases where correct procedures are used, and each progression fully established, one person is all that is necessary to handle a stroke patient. Where it is necessary to call in a second pair of hands it is wise to ask the question: 'Have correct procedures been followed step by step from the beginning?'

Figure 21 shows training of sitting balance. The patient's feet should be comfortably placed on the floor with both legs correctly positioned—that is, with knees apart and flexed to 90°, feet the same distance apart and parallel; thus the hip will be correctly positioned and external rotation will not be allowed. If the height of the bed is wrong and it cannot be adjusted, a wooden box or stool should be placed under the feet. (Polystyrene steps of different heights make a cheap and useful addition to physiotherapy equipment). Stabilising in sitting is routine physiotherapy and, in this case, it is a routine which must be carefully and thoroughly carried out. With sitting balance established, weight transference from hip to hip follows as a progression and next comes haunch walking forward to the edge of the bed (four small steps can usually be managed) and backward to the starting position. In each movement the hip must be lifted clear of the bed and the hands are clasped, palms touching, elbows extended. Alternatively, the arms may be placed at the patient's sides and the physiotherapist supports the affected arm as shown in Figure 23 or in Figure 7g. This means that the arm will be kept within the recovery pattern and weight bearing from elbow to shoulder, or from hand to shoulder, will be used. No opportunity to weight bear on the affected arm in the correct anti-spasm or recovery pattern must be neglected if arm rehabilitation is to be effective. To lift one hip clear of the bed, weight must be transferred laterally right across to the opposite side of the body. This exercise is stimulating tonic reflexes which produce involuntary changes in muscle tone in response to weight transference and head movements. In other words, this exercise is re-educating the postural reflex mechanism and at the same time inhibiting the dominating reflexes by careful positioning. The affected arm and leg are both clearly within the recovery pattern. Lateral transfers and haunch walking need not be fully established before the patient transfers to his chair. But this is an appropriate time to make a beginning in this very necessary exercise, and, therefore, this is an appropriate place in the text to point out the necessity for this important step in rehabilitation. The sooner lateral transfers are mastered the better, because they must be mastered if rehabilitation is to progress satisfactorily.

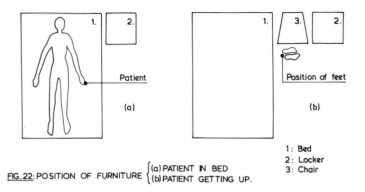

1 : Bed
2 : Locker
3 : Chair

FIG. 22: POSITION OF FURNITURE $\begin{cases} \text{(a) PATIENT IN BED} \\ \text{(b) PATIENT GETTING UP.} \end{cases}$

Figure 22 shows the correct positioning of ward furniture. We have already discovered the necessity to place the locker on the affected side when nursing the stroke patient. Difficulties which may include spatial orientation and/or neglect or denial of ownership of the affected side will be dealt with later when it is again found to be essential to have the locker on the affected side. Before the patient transfers to his chair, the chair must be placed as in Figure 22b. Handling the patient from the bed to the chair then becomes a quick, efficient action and gives the next progression in the total rehabilitation programme.

Figure 23 shows the transfer from bed to chair. This method of transfer is therapeutic as well as safe. The physiotherapist controls the patient's knees with her knees, she controls his forward lean to move his centre of gravity over his feet, she prevents internal rotation of the shoulder and she continues the programme of weight bearing from elbow to shoulder. Properly handled this method feels so safe to the patient it gives him confidence and the physiotherapist is in a position to ensure that her patient transfers part of his weight through his affected side. Correct positioning particularly of the arm must be maintained while the patient is taught to lean forward over his feet, to stand up, to give a quarter turn and sit down in the chair. The importance of placing the chair in the correct position before standing the patient will now be understood. Bare feet are an asset, stimulating sensation in the sole of the foot and holding the floor without slipping. However, if the floor is not suitably clean and the patient is diabetic, bare feet should not be allowed because of the danger of infection. In a later progression the patient should be taught to get up by himself. He should be taught to place his sound hand firmly on the bed and to lean on it while he stands, gives a quarter turn, and again leaning forward over his hand he places his buttocks backwards into the chair. Although this method may temporarily sacrifice lateral weight transference to the affected side, it gives the patient his first real step towards independence and, if it is correctly taught, it ought not to be a difficult progression and it ought to be achieved early in the rehabilitation programme.

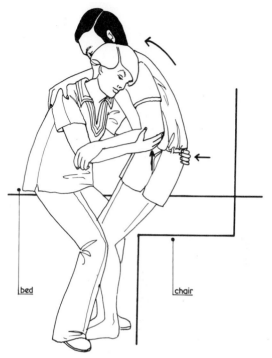

FIG.23:TRANSFER FROM BED TO CHAIR.

To help a patient to achieve even this small degree of independence as quickly as possible is to make a sound beginning towards helping him to overcome the disaster which has suddenly overtaken him and to make a start towards giving him back his self-respect.

The correct chair to be used must have a broad base, adequate armrests, and a seat at the right height to allow for sitting with the knees flexed to 90°. A further progression is made when the physiotherapist uses the handgrip illustrated in Figure 7g to assist her patient from the bed to the chair. This gives weight bearing from hand to shoulder and the movement again incorporates lateral transfer of body weight over the affected side when the patient makes the quarter turn to sit down. *A small table of adjustable height is used so that the patient may lean forward to support himself equally on both forearms with the forearms placed forward and parallel.* Lateral transference of weight from forearm to forearm should be practised in this position as a routine exercise and against resistance. The patient will be taught to make sure that the forearms do not turn inwards but point straight forward with wrist and fingers extended and thumb and fingers abducted. A brightly coloured stripe of Sellotape down the centre of the table will serve as a visual reminder to keep his forearms parallel. If the affected arm is

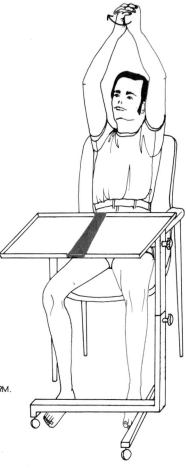

FIG. 24: SELF-CARE OF THE AFFECTED ARM.

allowed to turn inwards and the hand drifts across the coloured line, the shoulder will have moved into the forbidden spasm pattern of internal rotation.

Figure 24 shows self-care of the affected arm. The patient sits correctly positioned with the table in front of him and clasps his hands, palms touching, elbows extended, and maintains this position while he reaches both hands above his head to obtain shoulder protraction with external rotation and full elevation. If he looks up at his hands and rotates his forearms so that the affected arm turns into supination and the sound arm into pronation he will complete the anti-spasm pattern and neck extension will increase extensor tone in the affected forearm. This is an ideal self-care exercise for the following reasons:

1. It helps the patient to bring the affected hand into his mental picture of a whole body.

2. It helps him to be aware of its feel and of its position in space.

3. It works the affected arm in the full anti-spasm (or recovery) pattern and can be repeated by him many times a day.

4. It uses spinal reflexes to assist function and assists the main aim of re-establishing normal movement patterns while inhibiting developing spasticity.

5. As a self-care exercise it gives the patient the satisfaction of doing something useful for himself.

Arm elevation using two wooden handgrips fastened to a rope which is slung on an overhead pulley can only be of use *if* the patient is able to maintain external rotation of the affected shoulder. Further, the necessary use of a zipped flexion glove to ensure that the hand stays fixed to the pulley handle (or the need to bandage the hand into position) shows at a glance that the patient is not ready to maintain the position unaided. This condemns the practice outright. Without the patient's active assistance, the wooden handgrip will not maintain the affected arm in the anti-spasm pattern, nor will the exercise be truly self-care. For these reasons it is not advisable to use a pulley. With hands clasped, palms touching, the fingers are separated into abduction. If the thumb of the affected hand is uppermost it can be held in a good abduction position by the sound thumb. But many patients find it easier to feel what the affected hand is doing, and therefore to control it more easily, if the sound thumb is uppermost. It is senseless to destroy the patient's confidence and spoil the exercise by insisting that he places the affected thumb uppermost if he constantly gets it the other way round.

To get back into bed

To get back into bed the process described for getting out of bed is repeated in reverse. The patient stands, places his sound hand on the bed, takes a quarter turn to position his buttocks over the bed and sits down. From this sitting position he must not hook the sound leg under the affected leg to help it up onto the bed. Hooking, if it is allowed, will hold up normal development of controlled movement. He clasps his hands, palms touching, turns his head towards the foot of the bed and—extending his elbows—he swings both arms round to follow the movement of the head as he rolls back onto the bed, the sound leg following the trunk movement and the affected leg is supported, lifted, and swung into place on the bed by his helper. The sequence of movement is head, shoulders, arms, trunk rotation, legs—that is, the movement pattern is from head to foot in direction and so follows the normal sequence of movement in the development of purposeful, coordinated action—or controlled movement. This means that in the early days, however independently he may get out of bed, the nurse or physiotherapist must stand by to assist the patient's affected leg as he gets back into bed. This gives a very clear example of the way in which every activity of daily living from the onset of the stroke can be, and must be, incorporated into the treatment plan. This applies to the complete stroke who must be handled correctly in every detail from the day of onset. The aim is to give treatment of a very high standard, the object to rehabilitate a patient who will return to take up a normal life. On the other hand, it must not be forgotten that in all stroke rehabilitation, wherever possible, the method described for correct positioning and handling ought to be adopted for the patient's own physical and mental comfort and, hopefully, as a means of establishing some degree of self-care with independence as soon as possible.

Self-care

Self-care has a most important part to play in every stroke rehabilitation programme. Total independence is the aim of all treatment with a return to normal living. If this aim is to be achieved, or come anywhere near achievement, there must be no delay in starting activities in self-care. Rolling in bed, bridging, double arm elevation, rolling to reach for articles on a locker, rolling to sit up, sitting to standing and standing to sit on a waiting chair have all been shown as necessary steps in the rehabilitation programme and also as steps towards self-care. They are necessary steps in the rehabilitation programme because they use movement patterns that make it possible to begin the initial and very necessary early approach towards following the sequence of development as seen in the human infant: rolling → sitting → standing. The aim is to follow the development stages necessary to turn primitive reflex happenings into controlled movement where cortical restraint gives voluntary responses and learned skills. The patient has lost this ability on the affected side. A very sound beginning in his re-education has been made while preventive measures have been taken against developing spasticity by taking care to use the anti-spasm pattern and by diligent positioning at all times of resting. Rolling → propping → crawling → kneeling will come later in the physiotherapy department.

Also, early establishment of self-care exercise means that it will be possible for the patient himself to carry out the constant repetition of the movements necessary for recovery. So far it has been shown how the patient may very quickly learn to get himself out of bed using a therapeutic series of movements. It has been shown how he can cross facilitate by having a locker or table placed on his affected side, and again his movement keeps within the pattern for development of controlled movement. Finally the two most beneficial initial exercises he can use in the rehabilitation of his own arm by himself have been given— elbow propping and double arm elevation in the full anti-spasm pattern. This approach to treatment must surely show how wrong it is to stand over a struggling patient and insist that he dress himself, if, to do so, he is attempting an exercise that is far beyond his capability. Self-dressing will be incorporated in the self-care plan as early as possible; this means, as soon as it can be approached in a therapeutic way using the development patterns of movement in correct sequence. To allow a patient to use wrong movements which simply teach compensatory actions using the sound side of his body will interrupt the development pattern. Abnormal patterns of movement will be used, will be accepted by the brain, and it will later be impossible to get rid of them. This will effectively put an end to the aim of leading the patient back to total independence and a return to normal living. Worse still, excessive effort will lead to excessive stimulation of the unwanted reflexes.

When considering self-care it is important to remember:

1. Any activity given must be carefully assessed to make sure *the sequence of movement keeps within the development pattern:* e.g. placing the locker on the affected side ensures constant rolling across midline.

2. An area of ability is used to lead into any activity: e.g. *the eyes and head lead into rolling.*

3. *Each new position* that is reached in an advancing programme *must be carefully stabilised* before continuing.

4. *Constant repetition* must be given to make the relearning process possible and to speed up results.

5. *Assistance* with an exercise will lead to independence *but* an area of disability will not be expected to lead an activity *until muscle tone is returned to normal.*

6. It is most important to *avoid the frustration of failure.* Therefore, progress forward in the rehabilitation programme must be held within the patient's capability.

To sum up this chapter on the problem of developing spasm and the early treatment programme for the stroke patient, what is meant by the anti-spasm, or recovery, pattern has been shown. Each position that has been used and each exercise that has been given has kept well within this recovery pattern. Some very valuable conclusions have been reached and are listed below as a continuing guide to the reasoning behind this carefully planned rehabilitation programme.

Conclusions

1. The spasm pattern bears a direct relationship to the dominating reflexes.

2. The anti-spasm pattern is directly opposite to the spasm pattern.

3. The dominating reflexes are modified at cortical level when the postural reflex mechanism is fully established—in other words, when normal inhibiting influences have been restored, static reflexes once more become integrated into controlled movement.

4. All those who handle stroke patients must act as the inhibiting influence on the dominating reflexes (or developing spasm) until the postural reflex mechanism is fully established. This includes nurses, physiotherapists and occupational therapists.

5. This means that diligent positioning in the anti-spasm pattern must be maintained at all times and all exercise must work within this pattern. Also, all movements of the affected limbs will be assisted, or

active assisted movements, the operator maintaining the initiative and preventing the release of dominant reflex activity until static reflexes are integrated into controlled movement.

6. The correct sequence of controlled movement development closely follows the development patterns seen in the human infant as he rolls → sitting → standing, and as he rolls → propping → crawling → kneeling → standing.

7. Side-lying positions, which do not increase extensor tone, will be used wherever possible. Therefore, where it is necessary to increase extensor tone in the arm using the supine position, the legs will be positioned with extra care.

8. To teach the patient to compensate with his sound side is a disservice: e.g. to teach him to hook his sound foot under his affected foot to assist its movement is to teach him a habit which will ruin the correct sequence of controlled movement development and later pose very difficult problems.

9. Treatment must be early, intensive and repetitive if worthwhile results are to be obtained.

10. Self-care and all independent movement as given above, because it follows the sequence of motor development in the infant, and keeps well within the recovery pattern, does not lead to unwanted reflex activity.

11. Positioning in the spasm pattern, working into the spasm pattern, making excessive demands and encouraging early, willed, voluntary effort will all serve to stimulate unwanted dominant reflex activity and must be discarded from any treatment programme. *This means that the patient* **will not** *be asked to* **lead an activity with an area of disability until muscle tone is restored to normal:** e.g. he should not be allowed to use his hand in any way without forearm support until he can place his arm in space and hold it there.

3. Sensory loss

The problems of sensory loss

Sensory problems are by far the most difficult problems to overcome in stroke treatment, but, for all true rehabilitation, these problems must be overcome. A realistic approach to sensory loss and the difficulties that follow can only be made if the problems that present in our stroke patients are thoroughly understood. Hypertonicity has been discussed and the problem of spasm which commonly begins shortly after the onset of a stroke. It must be remembered that where spasticity is allowed to develop, within a year to eighteen months it will reach an extreme degree with the affected limbs held in total synergic patterns of tonic contraction which will successfully put an end to all worthwhile rehabilitation. Normal muscle tone has been discussed and accepted as entirely reflex in nature, anti-gravity muscles showing the greatest tone. The muscles are stretched between origin and insertion and the stretch stimulus initiates the reflex arc. In the stroke patient, if the reinforcing impulses from the vestibular nuclei are no longer inhibited from higher centres, it is reasonable to suppose and easy to accept the theory that all those who care for these patients must act as the missing and very necessary inhibiting influence on hypertonic, or increased, muscle tone. It has been shown how this may be done by careful positioning until the normal postural reflex mechanism is re-established and normal muscle tone restored. But, added to this, where necessary the physiotherapist must also find ways and means of *stepping up sensory input* to compensate for sensory loss.

When considering the sensory problems that may face the stroke patient it is necessary once again to go right back to the beginning and consider muscle tone. With stroke patients there will always be changes in muscle tone. These changes can be recognised in three ways which may present singly or, more usually, the changes will frequently overlap or co-exist. The clinical signs present as muscle spasm or spastic paralysis, as muscle weakness or flaccid paralysis, and as intention tremor with inability to hold a position in space, to overshoot in response to stimulation, or to drift when at rest. *Hypertonicity* = spasticity, and has been discussed. It is also necessary to consider the muscle weakness or flaccid paralysis which results from *hypotonicity* = reduced muscle tone. This leaves the patient with heavy 'rag-doll' limbs

43

which are quite unable to support him in the anti-gravity position on the affected side. Flaccid paralysis with these heavy, useless limbs is most marked where there is gross sensory loss.

If the spinal reflex arc (which maintains normal muscle tone) is broken by lesion of the motor nerves, of the sensory nerves or of the reflex centres, muscle tone will be lost. This is because the anterior horn of grey matter in the spinal cord contains vital cells which receive impulses from the proprioceptors along sensory neurones and from the motor area of the cerebral cortex. This means that the anterior horn cells relay voluntary movement impulses and they are also the motor neurones of the spinal reflex arc. Suppose, for example, the spinal reflex arc is broken by gross loss of proprioceptive sense, muscle tone will be lost. As *proprioceptive sense* is the sense of muscular position, or of muscle and joint position, with gross loss of this sense the stroke patient will no longer be aware of his position in space. *Anti-gravity and postural mechanisms,* therefore, are dependent on proprioceptive sense. Comprehension may be good, motor power intact, but *severe handicap will result and persist where this necessary factor is missing.* It must also be remembered that impulses set up by stimulation of proprioceptors in muscles, tendons and joints do not all end in the central nervous system controlling anti-gravity and postural mechanisms. In the normaily healthy body, a large number of these impulses also reach conscious-ness, travelling by afferent (sensory) pathways to the various internal structures of the brain which transmit information to the sensory receptive area of the cortex.

Damage to afferent pathways leads to problems of transmission within the brain (e.g. in the internal capsule) and to failure of the sensory receptive area to appreciate the stimulus. This gives paraesthesia or anaesthesia of cutaneous sensation and problems of spatial perception. Kinesthetic sense was described in Chapter 1. Failure to appreciate stimuli in the sensory receptive area will also mean that, with loss of receptive sensation, the patient will forget the feeling of normal move-ment; he will begin moving in abnormal patterns (where movement is possible) and he will very quickly memorise these abnormal movements and accept them as normal.

To touch briefly on other difficulties that may be encountered, deficit in the cortical sensory area may also include—with loss of cortical integration and sensory interpretation—a resulting loss of body image; the patient may no longer be aware of the affected half of his body, or, as might be expected, where the deficit is marked, he may not recognise the disability in the forgotten half. Such complex difficulties ought not to be allowed to confuse the issue; the outcome of the treatment programme must still be hopefully aimed at successful rehabilitation. Some phy-siotherapists tend to get lost in the jargon used to describe sensory problems and get no further than a half-hearted attempt to understand the words that are used.

A list of definitions of a few words that are most often used might be helpful here:

Agnosia: difficulty in recognition (here of half the body).

Anosognosia: failure to recognise the disability involving the forgotten half of the body, neglect or denial of ownership of the affected limbs.

Apraxia: a disturbance of visual-spatial relationships, or visual-spatial orientation which leads to inability to deal effectively with or manipulate objects, or to carry a task through.

Body image: body awareness, or the ability to feel a limb, to appreciate its place in space and its relationship to the rest of the body.

Hemianaesthesia: loss of sensation of the affected side.

Hemianopia: loss of the visual field on the affected side of the body.

Stereognosis: the recognition of familiar objects by their shape, size and texture when held in the hand with the eyes shut. (*Astereognosis* is sometimes used to describe failure to recognise familiar objects as above. Again it may be called *tactile agnosia*).

Spatial orientation: awareness of body position in relation to space.

I am convinced that if the physiotherapist is to make any sense of a plan to offer efficient rehabilitation to the stroke patient with sensory loss, she must approach the problem from the simple basic principle that all movement is a direct response to sensory stimuli from *vision, hearing, superficial pressure* and *deep pressure.* To make a beginning, from these sensory stimuli take one factor, proprioceptive sense—the sense of muscular position, or of muscle and joint position. Suppose, once more, that the spinal reflex arc is impaired by loss of proprioceptive sense, muscle tone is lost and the patient is no longer aware of the position in space of his affected limbs. I have said, if compensation for this missing factor is not made, severe handicap will persist and the patient's outlook will be dismal in the extreme with no prospect of anything like a return to normal living.

This looks a little like an insurmountable hurdle. We know if the *demand* (or sensory stimulation) from the higher centres of the brain is missing or impaired, it must be stepped up by adding stimuli from the proprioceptors, and, with increased *demand* a *response* will be gained. This must mean that with impaired proprioceptive sense there is vital sensory damage blocking the way to recovery. To add to the difficulty, re-education of the postural reflex mechanism depends on re-education from spinal reflex level, which will be much more demanding where there is loss of muscle tone because of interruption of reflex stimuli. The *demand* must be met and this can only be done by finding ways of stepping up the sensory input until a *response* is gained. Every means that can be devised to step up sensory input must be used.

It is proposed here to work out a reasoned and effective approach to the problem of rehabilitation of the stroke patient who has diminished, or missing, proprioceptive sense. A plan of treatment will be suggested and the patient will be offered a reasonable hope of recovery. It is a method of treatment which I have used over a period of ten years and it has given consistently good results.

Treatment plan for the stroke patient with sensory loss

Correct positioning and early handling of the stroke patient with sensory loss will be exactly the same as has already been given for the patient with hypertonicity and developing spasm. Sensory loss is often not detected in the very early days and, when it is found to be present, it will usually take time to identify the precise difficulty—particularly where dysphasia is an added complication. A short delay in reaching an accurate conclusion by careful assessment will not be important if correct handling with careful positioning has been instituted from the beginning. The essential point is to make an accurate assessment. Where there is sensory deficit *sensory input must be stepped up.* Also, where muscle tone is reduced to a state of flaccid paralysis, muscle tone must be increased by increasing the normal stimuli that maintain it. This involves repeated stretch, superficial and *deep pressure,* and weight-bearing through the limbs. So, once more, remembering that changes in muscle tone in the stroke patient frequently overlap and it will be uncertain in the early days which abnormal tone pattern will develop, correct positioning must be used as before and very carefully maintained.

I have chosen to illustrate this chapter on sensory loss by considering a patient who has *severe loss of proprioceptive sense* on his affected side. This has been chosen because it gives one of the very difficult problems in stroke rehabilitation and, if treatment is not effective, it leaves insoluble and permanent residual problems which cause great distress. In the past, the prognosis in this instance has been grave, the expectation of resuming anything like a normal life has been nil, and the patient has been faced with *severe and persistent handicap* with no hope of recovery. The lesion will be subcortical—between thalamus and cortex—and will involve postural sense or proprioceptive sense—the sense of muscular position, or muscle and joint position. We are here concerned with a servo mechanism—or a mechanism serving automatically to control the working of another mechanism. The servo system concerned in anti-gravity and postural mechanisms in the human body is dependent on proprioception. In other words, unless we can re-establish the missing sensory function our patient's severe handicap will persist.

The tests which are used to establish the state of the patient's postural sense are carried out—as might be expected—by flexing and extending his joints with his eyes closed. In the hand the index finger is used, in the foot the big toe. The patient is shown the movement and given the command: 'Look at your finger. It is up . . . it is down . . .' Then his eyes are covered and he is asked to state the position each time a move is made. If he is unsure or fails this test, we move up the limbs and test the larger joints. Grasping the thumb of the affected hand with the sound hand—eyes covered—is another test which may be used. The position of the affected arm is altered and the patient with defective proprioception will fail to find the thumb.

Supposing the patient has failed these tests, it will be necessary to plan a programme of treatment that will step up sensory input so that the prognosis for recovery need not and must not be poor. We must assess and reassess and plan and alter our programme accordingly, suiting the rehabilitation exercises to the age of the patient, the medical state of the patient, his exercise tolerance and his particular needs. But, for all patients with sensory loss, treatment is based on the following needs:

1. To increase muscle tone where necessary while at the same time insisting on careful positioning and use of the anti-spasm pattern.

2. To assess regularly so as to keep a careful eye on the state of muscle tone and to prevent any abnormal development of abnormal tonal patterns.

3. To *step up sensory input* so as to stimulate the reflex arc and reflex action, bombarding the proprioceptors with stimuli until we gain a response.

4. To stimulate anti-gravity and postural mechanisms, particularly by using approximation (or weight-bearing) to facilitate joint proprioceptors.

5. To re-educate controlled movement following the sequence of development as seen in the human infant, turning primitive reflex movement into purposeful, coordinated action.

Movement is a response to afferent information. Without adequate input, output will be inadequate. Without the knowledge of position in space it is not possible to move.

To step up sensory input

As already described, we use *hearing, vision* and *touch*.

Hearing: the commands given must be short, dynamic and delivered from the correct place to gain a response. Movement begins with the eyes which lead to turning the head. If the movement is to be to the right the physiotherapist will stand on the patient's right.

Vision: is used as above. The patient moves his eyes and turns his head to see the physiotherapist. Where the movement required is distal to proximal the patient may be firmly commanded to watch his hand or his foot. The use of a mirror will play a considerable part in rehabilitation. (Note that hemianopia will be dealt with later).

Touch: will play the biggest part in sensory re-education. When it is fully understood why touch must play the major role, it must then not be forgotten that vision and hearing must also be used as effectively as possible if the rehabilitation programme is going to be successful. *Touch must include* light pressure and *deep pressure.* If it does not include deep pressure sensory input is not being effectively stepped up and the rehabilitation effort will have a poor result.

To recapitulate: Pathways or nerve tracts in the spinal cord are *sensory* and *motor* and in the rehabilitation programme where we are dealing with *sensory* loss we are most concerned with *sensory* tracts.

The sensory nerve tract registers:

1. *Deep sensation:* which includes deep pain, *pressure* and the position of muscle and joint.

2. *Superficial sensation:* such as touch, pain, temperature and *pressure.*

Conclusion: We must use *deep pressure* to stimulate, or bombard, these sensory nerve-endings.

Author's note: I am presently treating an elderly lady of 82. After myocardial infarct three months ago she had a dense left-sided hemiplegia with severe hemianaesthesia. Joint and muscle sense on the affected side failed in all tests—large joints as well as small and she had a persistent and extreme degree of flaccidity or hypotonicity. After three months of intensive treatment she has re-established postural reflexes and redeveloped controlled movement. Her arm now has fully controlled shoulder movement against gravity and all her other arm movements—including pronation and supination—are present and controlled. Her hand movements are still weak but she has good opposition of thumb to fingers and she has begun to use the hand in free selective movements in the final sequence of distal to proximal. She is only one of the numbers who have made similar satisfactory progress and she is one of the many who must be offered a rehabilitation programme which will effectively step up sensory input to give a reasonable hope of a return to normal living. I said in the introduction that we have begun to ask the question, are we good enough? I would suggest now that if we are not offering this standard of rehabilitation, the answer must be no.

I propose to outline the treatment that can be offered to these patients

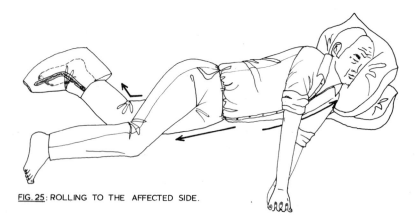

FIG. 25: ROLLING TO THE AFFECTED SIDE.

but, to save confusion, I will continue to assume that the patient is male and the physiotherapist female.

Rolling: will be carefully taught as before, but where there is sensory loss it is intensified to promote awareness of the affected side and to encourage normal limb movements. Techniques of treatment must once again be based on normal development of controlled movement as seen in the baby. The handclasp position—fingers interlaced, palms touching—will be actively encouraged. The aim is to help the affected side of the body to relate to the sound side. In the diagram, rolling to the affected side, Figure 25 shows correct positioning, trunk elongated by two pillows, hands clasped giving shoulder protraction with external rotation. The knee is flexed but the hip is shown in extension. This has been done to emphasise the need to keep a careful eye on hip extension—which must always be carefully watched in the early days in all patients because it is so easily lost. This is a very good resting position giving pressure on the affected side which assists the need for increased sensory input.

To roll on to the sound side as shown in Figure 26, the physiotherapist must step up sensory input by kneeling or standing beside her patient's sound side and giving a firm command so that he will turn his eyes, his head and, maintaining the handclasp position, swing his arms across midline to his sound side. Assistance in making full use of the resulting trunk rotation to give a follow-through of leg movement may be given by the physiotherapist in the early days of treatment. She places her

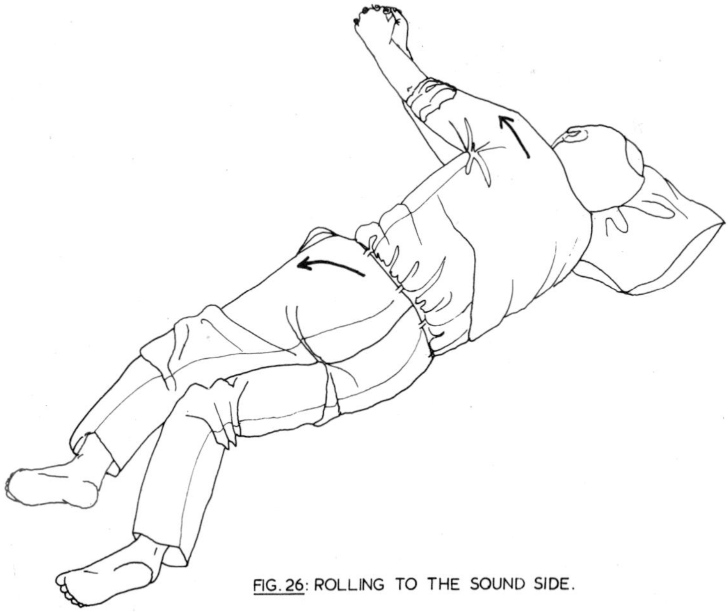

FIG. 26: ROLLING TO THE SOUND SIDE.

hand in a suitable position to assist pelvic roll with protraction and the leg follows. Again this is a good resting position but because of resulting pressure, lying on the affected side is of greater value where there is sensory loss.

Notice in Figures 25 and 26, bearing in mind the necessity to watch the position of the trunk, the patient rolls on to two pillows on the affected side, one on the sound side. Care must be taken not to trap the affected shoulder in a bad position under the body when rolling to the affected side. This will not happen if the correct handclasp position is used and the shoulders held well forward in protraction. Both of these good resting positions should be used frequently during treatment sessions. This means that the elderly, frail patient is able to tolerate the intensive, repetitive treatment necessary for recovery because exercise will be liberally punctuated with resting periods in therapeutic positions. Again, bearing in mind what has already been said about the need to maintain and work into the recovery pattern at all times, these two diagrams serve as a reminder that positioning is not at any time forgotten or left out of the scheme of the careful rehabilitation pro-gramme. Handled like this, correct positioning is very quickly esta-blished and at no time forgotten by the physiotherapist—and usually by the patient who will frequently maintain correct positions and practise correct movements without being told.

Bridging: will be carefully taught for the same reasons as before, care being taken to ensure that the correct starting position has been stabilised and firmly established. Where the patient shows a tendency to allow the affected leg to fall or to drift into external rotation at the hip, a brisk tapping on the internal femoral condyle of the affected leg will give an effective sensory reminder. Placing a hard-backed book between the knees can also be very effective. The patient is taught to watch the book, to press both knees firmly against it to hold it in position and to maintain his hold with the knees pointing to the ceiling (or mildly rotated to the sound side) for as long as possible. Competition between patients in this exercise always stimulates lively interest and can add the final step up in demand to gain the required response. This can lead fairly quickly into control of hip rotation.

Rolling to elbow propping: or side lying with elbow support, must be established as soon as possible—if this has not already been achieved in bed exercise. It is an essential exercise, particularly where there is sensory loss and the very urgent need for early weight-bearing from elbow to shoulder. But, with sensory loss, it is more difficult to establish. The physiotherapist will hold the affected arm in position. In a left-sided stroke she holds the affected forearm firmly in position with her left hand and physiotherapist and patient take a handshake grasp with their right hands to assist his roll forwards and sideways into elbow propping. The elbow is well forward, shoulder protracted in a good position, and the patient is taught to balance over the affected forearm. Assistance will

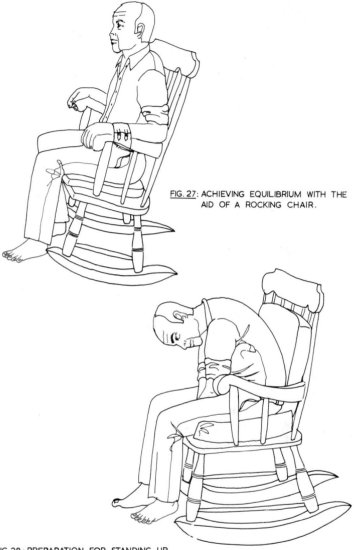

FIG. 27: ACHIEVING EQUILIBRIUM WITH THE AID OF A ROCKING CHAIR.

FIG. 28: PREPARATION FOR STANDING UP.

be given in maintaining the position where necessary, then it will be stabilised and a later progression will be made when it is held against resistance.

A rocking chair ought to be used. It is an invaluable aid in all stroke rehabilitation. In Figure 27 the patient is using the almost spontaneous movement that results from sitting in a rocking chair. He begins by gentle rocking, pushing on the sound foot. Pushing on both feet quickly follows, leading to hip and trunk flexion and extension with pressure on the forearms, and neck reflexes are stimulated. Elderly patients usually take to a rocking chair like ducks to water. Stabilising in sitting and re-education of postural reflexes quietly moves forward and is frequently rapidly established with little effort and no frustration. A quiet contentment is often noticed. Rocking to suitable music is a favourite exercise. Again the limbs are carefully positioned. The starting position has hips and knees flexed to 90°, knees apart and directly above the feet and the affected hip is not allowed to drift or fall into external rotation. Pressure on the foot *must* pass through the heel. I frequently use a foot 'rest' cut deeply into thick foam rubber so that pressure can only take place through the heel while the forepart of the foot is unsupported in space. This thick block of foam rubber also greatly assists correct foot positioning. The arm is not allowed to hang from the shoulder in internal rotation. Leaning forward with clasped hands, elbows extended (Fig. 28), is taught in preparation for standing up. Bare feet will help to boost sensory input. Remember the need for extra care in hygiene if the patient is diabetic.

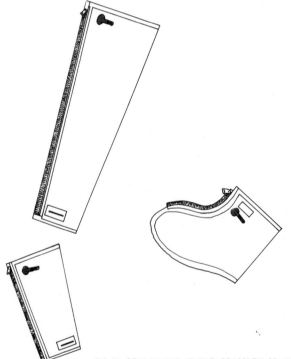

FIG. 29: ORALLY INFLATABLE PRESSURE SPLINTS-
AN AID TO REHABILITATION.

It will now be understood that the rehabilitation programme has continued, moving forward from ward level to the physiotherapy department, with exercises that are common to all stroke patients whether or not the patient shows sensory loss. I have simply pointed out some factors in the rehabilitation programme that boost sensory input. For successful rehabilitation there will be many cases where this is not adequate. To gain the required degree of success in the patient with severe hemianaesthesia it is urgently necessary to find a way of introducing far greater sensory stimuli. Otherwise rehabilitation efforts are doomed to failure. Very briefly, let me present the case for the use of pressure splints in the treatment of stroke patients.

The use of pressure splints

Ten years ago, while attempting to find an answer to the residual problem of the hemiplegic arm, I began using the inflatable pressure splint. An orally inflatable arm splint, made of clear plastic casing forming a double sleeve, came into my possession quite by chance. I saw at once that, when the splint was fitted to the arm and fully inflated orally, pneumatic cushioning conformed to the shape of the limb, holding it immobile and suspended to give full support with all over *even pressure*. The splint is X-ray transparent and was designed as an emergency splint for first-aid and safe transport of fractured, crushed or sprained limbs (Fig. 29). It seemed to me that the splint ought to provide the necessary missing support and sensory stimulation to assist my attempt to find a way round the problems that prevented recovery in so many stroke patients. As shown in Figure 29, the splint represented is a United States patent. For information on available sources of supply turn to the end of the book.

The main problems in order of difficulty were:
1. Sensory loss
2. Severe hypotonicity (or flaccidity)
3. A developing (or advanced) state of hypertonicity (or spasticity)

Application of the splint:
The pressure splint was applied with the shoulder in external rotation and with elbow, wrist and fingers in extension and the thumb in abduction. That is, the arm was held fully in the recovery pattern.

Sensory loss:
The pressure splint, in this instance, is used to apply even deep pressure to the soft tissues. With the demand from the higher centres of the brain missing, or impaired, it must be stepped up by bombarding the proprioceptors with stimuli and, with this increased demand a response is gained. With diminished proprioceptive sense there is a tremendous hurdle blocking recovery—but the pressure splint offered a way over the hurdle. The demand must be placed where the response is required. The

sensory nerve tract registers *deep sensation* which includes pressure and the position of muscle and joint (or proprioceptive sense). If sensory input must be stepped up sufficiently to gain a response and proprioceptive sense is diminished, it seemed to me that the pressure splint offered the missing link in stroke rehabilitation. In this instance sensory input can only be stepped up satisfactorily by applying sufficient pressure to stimulate deep sensation. All stroke rehabilitation works from the spinal reflex level upwards until cortical level is re-established and bombardment of proprioceptors must be used to activate the anterior horn cell. Exercise gives movement within the tissues and exercise given under pressure must be more effective.

Severe hypotonicity (or flaccidity)

The pressure splint offered the necessary supporting assistance to make it possible for the physiotherapist to give the essential exercise techniques which must include the heavy compression force of approximation—or weight bearing through a correctly positioned limb in order to stimulate underlying postural reactions, **including joint proprioceptors,** and further boost defective afferent information.

A developing hypertonicity (or spasticity)

The pressure splint held the limb in the full recovery pattern. In other words it inhibited dominant reflexes and it was found that treatment with the splint reduced spasticity dramatically and made re-education possible. Where finger spasm had been allowed to develop, making it difficult to apply the splint, it was found that brisk tapping or pounding on the proximal part of the palm of the hand made it possible to apply the splint with the hand in the recovery (anti-spasm) pattern.

In the rehabilitation programme, where there is gross sensory loss and sensory nerves accommodate to sustained pressure, *intermittent pressure* may also be used to give movement within the tissues and a satisfactory answer to the need to boost proprioceptive sense still further. A mechanical pump supplies intermittent and controlled pneumatic pressure and may be safely applied to arm or leg. There are various pumps on the market. I have used the American Jobst Extremity Pump and the British Flowtron System. The British pump has proved efficient and much less costly. Also, the arm sleeves supplied with this pump are open-ended which makes for easy application and, as intermittent pressure sleeves are not transparent, allows for checking the correct positioning of hand and arm with external rotation of the shoulder. Where it is necessary to include intermittent pressure in the treatment programme because of gross loss of proprioceptive sense, I give a daily session of at least one hour using the Flowtron System. For the limb of average girth I turn the pressure control to No. 8—using 7 for a swollen or larger limb—and the arm is very carefully positioned in elevation with external rotation of the shoulder. The results I have obtained have been most satisfactory.

Note: This type of mechanical intermittent pressure should not be used on patients in acute pulmonary oedema and should be used with caution on those with congestive heart failure or in those where pre-existing deep vein thrombosis is suspected. Where a compression boot is used on the lower leg it is easy to position the leg correctly; where the longer full leg sleeve is used special care must be taken to maintain the leg in slight elevation with the hip in internal rotation. The use of an intermittent pressure pump does not mean that the orally inflated splint can be dispensed with. It *must* be applied and used during treatment sessions in the series of exercises which involve the careful techniques necessary to promote recovery.

Figure 30a, b, c shows the correct application of the arm splint. *Figure 31* shows a patient suitably positioned while at rest with the splint in place. The points to note are:

1. The arm is in elevation and external rotation.
2. The affected leg is carefully positioned.
3. The neck is carefully positioned to increase extensor tone in the forearm.
4. Increased extensor tone in the shoulder is counteracted by the arm positioning in elevation.

NOTE: The shoulder <u>must</u> be externally rotated.

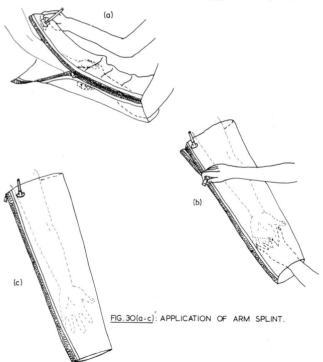

FIG. 30(a-c): APPLICATION OF ARM SPLINT.

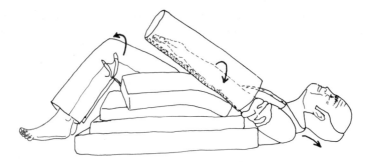

FIG. 31 : ARM ELEVATION WITH PRESSURE SPLINT.

5. Where the splint is used to counteract developing spasm it is used in preference to the intermittent pressure splint because it holds the limb firmly in the anti-spasm pattern. The key points of spasm control in the arm are neck, upper spine, shoulder girdle, wrist and fingers. With the positioning described above, and the addition of the orally inflated splint to maintain the extended wrist, abducted fingers and finger-tip pressure, all key points are activated simultaneously. Hence the immediate comfort the splint gives with quite spectacular control of any spastic resistance. This can be quite dramatic in a patient who has been badly handled and is beginning to produce the painful shoulder syndrome.

If the treatment session begins with mat work—positioning, rolling, bridging and hip rotation—a suitable rest period may be introduced while pressure treatment is given to the affected arm. Treatment is comfortable and, as long as careful positioning is used, it is a thoroughly therapeutic resting exercise and the patient frequently falls asleep. A session in pressure treatment begins:

(a) with intermittent pressure, or

(b) without intermittent pressure.

(a) Where developing spasm is minimal or absent, and sensory loss is present, the intermittent pump is used for a session of at least half an hour. As soon as the arm sleeve is removed, the arm exercises as already used in the ward (Figs. 14, 15 and 16) are given. Then the orally inflatable splint is applied and pressure treatment resumed by giving a resting period of at least half an hour, as in Figure 31, followed by an exercise session with the splint in place.

Where sensory loss in the leg causes severe problems, intermittent pressure to the leg will be used. In this case the patient is positioned lying on his sound side and the affected limbs are supported on pillows. For exercise periods an orally inflated pressure boot—or foot and ankle splint—can be useful as a treatment aid.

(b) Where sensory loss is not the problem and pressure is being used as the inhibiting influence on hypertonic motor neurones (or developing spasm) until the missing postural reflex mechanism is re-established and normal inhibiting influences restored, intermittent pressure is not used. In this case the orally inflatable splint is applied and the resting period of half an hour is given as in Figure 31. This is followed by the exercise session with the splint still in place. Where sustained pressure is used only orally inflated splints are suitable. This is because the warmth of the breath makes the inner plastic sheath pliable so that it moulds satisfactorily to the limb to give an all over even pressure without severe compression. To achieve satisfactory results the splint ought to be fully inflated and it must be correctly applied to give full stretch into the inhibiting position, thus gaining an additional boost to recovery by activating the Golgi organs.

It now becomes reasonably clear that it is impossible to divide the treatment programme into two distinct fields, one dealing with the problem of developing spasticity and the other dealing with the problem of sensory loss. Both are motor problems and, therefore, inseparable. While considering one of the most serious problems sensory loss can represent (loss of proprioceptive sense) it has been seen that methods used for stepping up sensory input also assist in inhibiting dominant reflexes. This should not be surprising as rehabilitation for all stroke patients is concerned with re-establishing postural reflexes and developing controlled movement in response to reflex activity. If motor loss is complicated by sensory loss this does not alter the rehabilitation programme. but it does mean that careful thought must be given to the urgent need to step up sensory input. It may also be necessary to use careful techniques to increase muscle tone where flaccidity is the problem and this factor pinpoints the need for regular and careful assessment to establish the individual tonal pattern. As described above, the pressure splint serves a triple purpose. It stimulates sensory nerve endings registering deep pressure and the position of muscle and joint, it offers supporting assistance for necessary exercise sessions and it inhibits dominating reflexes.

It is proposed to continue the rehabilitation programme by laying down a broad plan for successful treatment. *Motor development and sensory development progress together* **but** the state of muscle tone found to be present will dictate the finer adjustments to be made to the broad plan. No two patients are exactly the same; symptoms must be assessed and re-assessed and treatment offered according to the findings.

Conclusion

Where severe handicap is present because the servo system concerned in anti-gravity and postural mechanisms lacks proprioception, the pressure splint may be used to supply the necessary force to bridge the gap. It is necessary to work out a pressure splint procedure—or specialised techniques—that will assist the splint to become an effective tool to be used in this way. It should also be remembered that, as well as inhibiting dominant reflexes by holding the arm in the recovery pattern, stimulation of the Golgi organs (or specialised proprioceptors in the musculo-cutaneous junctions) is obtained and these are receptive to stretch, having an inhibitory effect on motoneurone pools of their own muscle supply.

4. Broad treatment plan

Pressure splint procedure

There is a place for deep pressure therapy in the treatment of all stroke patients because there is always a disturbance of normal tone and there is usually a need to step up sensory input. Accordingly, deep pressure therapy will be included as a necessary and integral part of complete treatment. The splint is applied as shown in Figures 30 and 31 and treatment begins with a resting period of at least 20 minutes. An exercise session follows. The exercises will be chosen and graded to suit the individual patient.

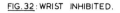
FIG. 32 : WRIST INHIBITED.

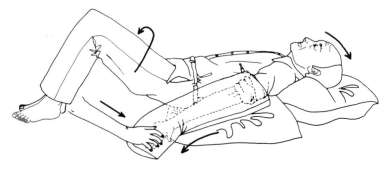

Figure 32 shows the inhibited wrist with a pressure splint in place. The physiotherapist works from the patient's affected side. The artist's diagram does not give the double handgrip that is used to give approximation with the shoulder suitably supported. This has been done in order not to obstruct the clear view of the patient's position. The dominating reflexes give wrist flexion and it is most important to prevent the stiff, flexed wrist that so frequently develops where treatment is neglected. Where this is allowed to happen it effectively prevents the necessary approximation or *weight-bearing, from the proximal part of the palm of the hand to the shoulder which is an essential feature of all worthwhile treatment. The pressure splint is used to simulate and produce the same effects as weight-bearing, giving postural fixation with sensory stimulation, allowing the necessary weight-bearing to be*

undertaken. This means that the physiotherapist gives approximation from the heel of the hand to the shoulder through an extended elbow with the shoulder in external rotation. The inhibited wrist position is used from the earliest days of treatment and, if correct handling has been followed, with the pressure splint in place it is pain free. Approximation from heel of hand to shoulder will be given with counter-pressure from the shoulder which is held in protraction with external rotation. The physiotherapist will find she needs two hand holds for both of these exercises, firstly to assist in supporting the splint while she obtains good wrist extension and, secondly, to support the shoulder correctly and give counter-pressure for approximation. A half arm splint is suitable provided it supports the elbow well. A full arm splint ought to be used for the patient with long arms.

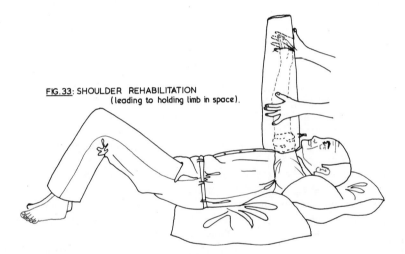

FIG. 33: SHOULDER REHABILITATION
(leading to holding limb in space).

Figure 33 shows shoulder rehabilitation—arm elevation in external rotation. With the pressure splint on, this exercise is established early as an active assisted exercise. Where hypertonicity is the problem, mobility of the shoulder girdle is noticeably facilitated where spastic resistance of the scapula muscles is at its lowest with the pressure splint on.

With hypertonicity (spasticity) there is loss of movement with loss of rotation and *the aim is to mobilise into external rotation and encourage movement.* Extra care in preventing a drift into the tonic synergic pattern of internal rotation of the shoulder must always be taken where there is hypertonicity and this is combined with re-education from passive to assisted to active assisted movement and the ability to place and hold the arm in space without drifting into internal rotation. The use of the pressure splint, correctly applied so as to inhibit the spasm pattern, removes the impediments in the way of successful rehabilitation and greatly assists *the aim of mobilising the shoulder into external rotation and encouraging normal movement patterns.*

With hypotonicity (flaccidity) there is flaccid loss of movement with resulting loss of stability and *the aim is to stabilise joints and mobilise into movement* by making an increased sensory demand (particularly on joint proprioceptors). Where proprioceptive sense is impaired there is an urgent need to step up sensory stimulation. The increased sensory demand made by the pressure splint on muscles and joints by deep pressure and the support which helps to simulate weight-bearing and assist in techniques of approximation greatly assists *the aim of stabilising and mobilising into movement.*

As I have said, tonal patterns frequently overlap and co-exist; the skill of the physiotherapist must be used to make an accurate assessment of the symptoms and to treat accordingly. The common factor in rehabilitation treatment, whatever the change in muscle tone, is the need to mobilise into movement. This aim will be achieved if extra care in preventing drift into the tonic synergic pattern of rotation is taken where there is hypertonicity, and extra care in stabilising is taken where there is hypotonicity.

In arm elevation in external rotation (Fig. 33), where hypertonicity is the main problem, the arm is held fully in the anti-spasm pattern and movement is encouraged in the anti-spasm or recovery pattern. In the early stages of rehabilitation the weight of the splint will be held and guided by the physiotherapist who maintains the initiative. This active assisted movement leads to placing the limb against gravity in space and holding it there—or to 'placing' and 'holding'. The stability of holding the limb in space is necessary before purposeful movement can be achieved. As soon as sustained holding is established active movement begins. One stage leads to the next, no stage can be omitted, but where the splint is used the rehabilitation time is considerably lessened. Where there is hypotonicity the splint adds the stability that is frequently impossible to establish without this aid and it also makes it possible to apply the necessary approximation to stabilise the shoulder. Approximation encourages the deficient extrapyramidal activity and stimulates flaccid shoulder muscles by producing co-contraction of the muscles round the joint. Proprioceptive sense is given a dynamic boost.

These introductory notes on the active use of the pressure splint should make it quite clear that this aid to treatment is of great value for all stroke rehabilitation.

Note: This is an appropriate place to remember two points:

1. Internal rotation of the shoulder and external rotation of the hip are the positions the shoulder and hip joints drift into with tonic contraction. Therefore, the shoulder is mobilised into external rotation, the hip into internal rotation. This is the key to all correct positioning and the basic fact to remember so that all rehabilitation leads into the anti-spasm or recovery pattern.

FIG. 34: SHOULDER PROTRACTION, WRIST INHIBITED.

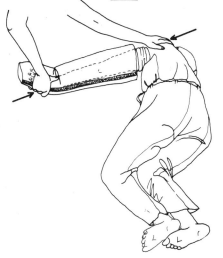

2. Where arm rehabilitation is carried out in supine lying (the position which builds up extensor spasm) the leg must always be carefully positioned in the anti-spasm or recovery pattern.

Figure 34 shows shoulder protraction, wrist inhibited. This is an essential early exercise and the diagram shows correct positioning. The patient lies on his sound side and the physiotherapist has full control of the arm with the assistance of the splint. She places one hand over the scapula and she must make sure that the movement is not a roll. Firm balance in side-lying has been established and the movement takes place in the shoulder-girdle, the scapula moving round the chest wall. Clear instruction ought to be given to the patient. He is asked to maintain the side-lying position and not to roll and he is told that the movement will take place only in the shoulder. 'I want you to help me to reach your arm forward . . . and back again . . .' A freely mobile scapula is essential to shoulder mobilisation. *Approximation is also practised in this position, the physiotherapist's handgrips being used to support and give counter-pressure.* Where an assistant is available, the tonic neck reflex may be incorporated to advantage. The patient's head is placed with his neck in extension with rotation to the affected side and he is asked to hold this position against resistance. This brings in the asymmetrical neck extension response to increase extensor tone in the affected arm. Arm elevation with external rotation may also be practised while lying on the sound side.

Figure 35 shows the arms correctly positioned while hip rotation is practised. The sound arm is stretched forward and the hands are held palm to palm, both pressing against the splint to help to maintain

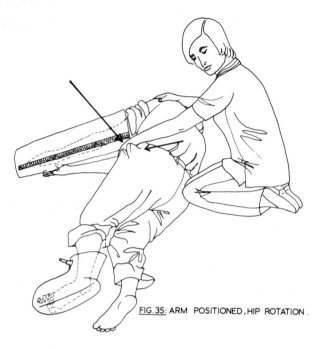

FIG.35: ARM POSITIONED, HIP ROTATION .

contact between the sound side and the affected side. Inability to feel the affected arm, or to appreciate its place in space or its relationship to the rest of the body demonstrates as loss of body image. As used here, the pressure splint will have a positive effect on loss of body image. The physiotherapist gives a supporting hold over the affected shoulder and alters the position of her second hand, moving it backward and forward from the anterior aspect of the iliac crest to the posterior aspect to give an active assisted movement which includes lower trunk rotation, pelvic rotation and hip flexion and extension. Resisted movements follow as a progression. Trunk movements are established first and hip control *must* be established in the early days. **Successful rehabilitation depends on establishing hip and shoulder control early in the treatment programme.** The necessary first step has been taken by establishing early and correct positioning of the hip and shoulder, the second step must be the development of controlled movement in these two vital joints. Without this concept of treatment, and with failure to take these two necessary first steps in rehabilitation, the treatment programme will fail before it begins. Therefore, upper trunk rotation will also be given with the patient lying on his sound side as in Figure 35. A pillow may be placed between the arms to support the pressure splint and give a friction free surface. The splint will slide forward and backward while the exercise is repeated at shoulder level, movement taking place in the upper trunk and shoulder while the lower trunk is held immobile. With the pressure splint in place there is no danger of any undesirable effect from irradiation (or overflow of activity) into the arm. Remembering that early trunk rotation from supine to prone is a mass flexion pattern, forward rotation against resistance might, for example, stimulate unwanted forearm flexion into the spasm pattern *but* the splint would then trigger off one of the key points of spasm control—the finger-tips. Note that the pressure boot can be very useful as an aid to treatment where extra sensory stimulation is needed and it holds the ankle in the anti-spasm pattern. Again, all over even pressure does not produce unwanted reflex activity.

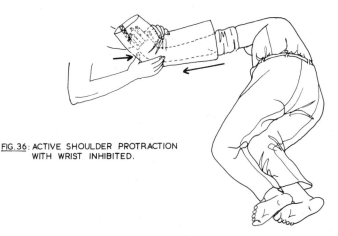

FIG.36: ACTIVE SHOULDER PROTRACTION WITH WRIST INHIBITED.

Figure 36 shows a further progression in shoulder rehabilitation— active protraction with the wrist inhibited. Active upper trunk rotation may also be practised with the physiotherapist in this position. This time the patient is asked to roll his upper trunk and he is taught to lead the movement with his eyes and head. The physiotherapist goes with the movement, supporting and guiding the splint and later resistance may be added. Again, it must be remembered, it also gives a very suitable position for an assistant to give neck extension with lateral flexion to the affected side against resistance plus counter-pressure on the affected shoulder, while the essential exercise of approximation from the heel of the hand to the shoulder is given.

Figure 37 shows the application of a hand and wrist splint so that shoulder elevation with a flexed elbow may be practised. This facilitates shoulder movement by shortening the lever. All the beginning arm movements are initially assisted with the physiotherapist maintaining the initiative. The limb must be able to *place* and *hold* in space before active movements begin. The same rule applies to the leg but our past very poor rate of success in arm rehabilitation has frequently been because this rule has been ignored. Again this comes back to the

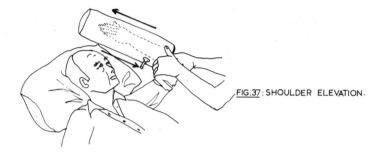

FIG.37 : SHOULDER ELEVATION.

essential factor—controlled movement must be developed in the shoulder and hip before making any attempt to establish controlled movement in the elbow, hand, knee and foot. In this instance, as soon as controlled shoulder movement is gained, the physiotherapy treatment programme will move on to active and then to resisted movement. It is essential to give correct patterns of movement and not to let the limb drift into the pattern of spasticity. The patient must not be allowed to develop wrong and trick movements which he will establish in his memory bank and fail to discard later e.g. shoulder elevation is not achieved by lateral flexion of the trunk.

Figure 38 showing early elbow rehabilitation, emphasises the point that it is necessary for the patient to maintain, establish or re-educate the feel of normal movement while he stays within the recovery pattern. Assisted elbow flexion and extension may be practised as in Figure 38, the physiotherapist asking the patient to assist the movement. He is encouraged to use his eyes and the commands that are given are simple and dynamic. 'Look at your hand. Take your hand down to your face . . . Now help me to lift it up again . . .' While practising this exercise the physiotherapist alters her right hand hold to give maximum proprio-

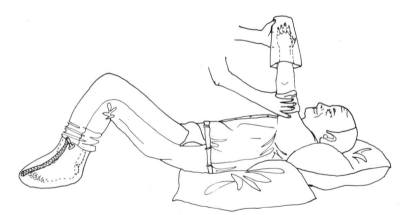

FIG.38: ELBOW REHABILITATION.

ceptive stimulation. As illustrated in Figure 38, pressure over triceps is being given to assist extension of the elbow. 'Look at your hand . . . Now help me to lift it towards the ceiling . . .' and, with this command, pressure is applied over the triceps. The correct manual contacts to gain the required response must always be taken into account.

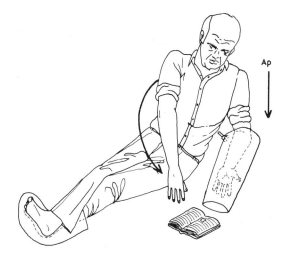

FIG.39: ELBOW PROPPING : CROSS FACILITATION.

Figure 39 shows elbow propping in an exercise in cross facilitation. Notice that the sound leg rolls over the affected leg. If rolling and rolling to elbow propping have been carefully established in the early and correct sequence of rehabilitation, this exercise will not pose any problems. It is a useful position to adopt when the coffee or tea break interrupts the treatment session. Where it will be understood, and this includes the majority of patients, it is best to explain why an exercise is carried out, what it will do to help recovery and why it must be carefully and correctly done. When the rehabilitation programme has progressed this far the patient is frequently carefully maintaining his own correct positioning and it becomes automatic *if* it has been diligently pursued from the day of onset of the stroke. Elbow propping, as in Figure 39, is a thoroughly therapeutic exercise, the sound side of the body working across midline to the affected side. A block of sorbo rubber eight or ten inches square under the lateral aspect of the affected hip is a suitable aid towards maintenance of good internal rotation of the affected hip. The trunk is elongated on the affected side, approximation takes place from elbow to shoulder and once the position is firmly established it will be cheerfully maintained for coffee break. Note: Rolling to elbow propping is a component of the righting response that must be re-educated and leads to sitting and the ability to sit upright. Therefore, this exercise is re-

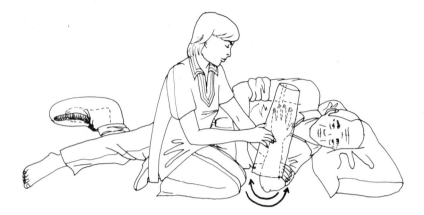

FIG.40: LYING ON AFFECTED SIDE ELBOW AND HIP REHABILITATION.

educating the ability to hold the upright position, improving body image and re-educating lost shoulder function.

Figure 40 shows elbow and hip rehabilitation while the patient lies on his affected side. Remembering that hip extension must not be lost, the affected hip is fully extended and the knee flexed. A pressure boot very often helps to establish and maintain this leg position. Lying on the affected side assists in sensory stimulation. It must be remembered that the patient must only roll on to a shoulder that is well forward in protraction; he must not be allowed to roll on to a retracted shoulder that will be trapped below him. He learns to roll with extended elbows and will usually support the splint with his sound hand. Again, while exercising the elbow, he is told to watch his hand and to follow the movement with his eyes. Flexion against gravity and extension against mild resistance will begin as soon as assessment shows that the patient is ready to make the progression. He is taught to keep his palm turned towards his face, staying out of the pattern of forearm pronation.

Continuing redevelopment of normal movement

These pressure splint exercises for the affected arm make a sound beginning towards efficient and functional rehabilitation of the arm and, at the same time, serve to show that at no time in the treatment programme is functional rehabilitation of the leg neglected or forgotten. Recovery of controlled movement in the shoulder and hip must proceed together. Correct positioning has been maintained throughout, proprioceptors have been bombarded to step up sensory input and, where there is marked loss of proprioceptive sense it has been shown that approximation must be intensified. All the exercises are very important, but the notes that are given for Figures 30 to 33 should be understood and the correct progression will then be made. It is important to note that the splints are applied with the hand far enough back from the open end to maintain pressure on the finger-tips. The splint should extend well above the elbow except where the exercise includes elbow flexion. Early weight-bearing through an extended elbow from the heel of the hand to the externally rotated shoulder is of prime importance. The splints will be removed and re-applied during the treatment session and an exercise that is achieved with the splint on will be attempted with the splint off— provided the physiotherapist retains the initiative and does not allow irradiation to stimulate the undesired spasm pattern. All progressions will be made as a result of careful assessment. Frequent short rolling sessions will punctuate the treatment routine, as will bridging to assist in establishing controlled hip extension and early weight-bearing. At all times the patient's tolerance to exercise must be taken into account. To obtain the maximum deep pressure effect, and therefore the maximum benefit, the orally inflated splint must be applied with the maximum pressure the human lungs can give.

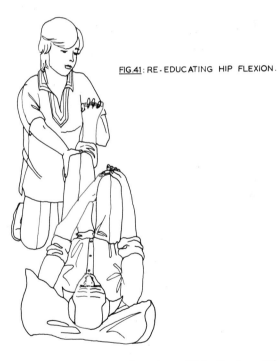

FIG.41: RE-EDUCATING HIP FLEXION.

Figure 41 shows further re-education of hip flexion. Hip flexion is facilitated by using flexion of the sound leg to tilt the pelvis. The patient is taught to clasp his hands and hold them round the sound knee as in the diagram. The patient's handclasp position holds the affected arm out of the forbidden spasm pattern and assists in re-education of missing body image, keeping the affected arm always in mind and in his mental picture of a whole body. Flexion of the affected hip is then taught, working through the stages of assisted active movement, to placing the limb with the knee at 90°, as in the diagram, to holding in this position, to active controlled movement. When holding the limb as in the diagram, approximation may be applied from knee to hip to advantage. If the hip tends to drift into external rotation, the physiotherapist will facilitate internal rotation and active holding of the limb in space if she maintains her handgrip on the toes and uses her other hand to give short, brisk tapping to the medial aspect of the knee joint. For resting periods the legs return to the crook position as taught for bridging. If the resting position is to be held for any length of time, correct positioning of pillows will assist shoulder and hip protraction. The patient may be asked to hold a book between his knees while he rests. This gives a visual reminder that the knees are to be kept together in mid-position and the affected knee must not be allowed to drift, giving external rotation of the hip. The book also gives a sensory reminder through touch (or pressure) on the inner or medial aspect of the knee joint. With the book still in position he may be asked to rotate his hips slightly towards the sound side. This is an excellent resting position and, at the same time, maintaining it correctly helps to establish hip control. It must not be forgotten that supine lying is the position which produces maximal extensor spasticity and where supine lying is used diligent positioning must be maintained. For lengthy resting periods side lying will be used.

Figure 42 shows the patient learning to establish controlled hip rotation by abduction and adduction of the knee, as distinct from the mild hip rotation that occurs together with hip flexion and extension as shown in Figure 35. This exercise must follow the hip, pelvic and lower trunk rotation as demonstrated in Figure 35 if full hip control is to be established. The illustration (Fig. 42) also shows what will happen if the physiotherapist gives resisted movement before assessment shows that the patient is ready for it. The effort involved in trying to hold internal rotation against resistance is producing irradiation, or overflow of movement, into the affected arm and the arm position is moving into forearm flexion with supination and internal rotation of the shoulder. Recovery will be aided in this situation if a pressure splint is placed on the arm and the anti-spasm pattern fully maintained *but* this will be done only after the initial early training. It will first be necessary to follow the correct sequence of rehabilitation to re-educate the ability to sustain posture. It is always necessary to move through the stages of passive movement to assisted movement, to active assisted movement, to placing and holding in space, to controlled movement. Where necessary muscle tone will be increased by brisk tapping (or prodding with the finger-tips) as above, by deep pressure and by approximation of joint surfaces. In the jargon of the physiotherapist, 'the stability of sustained posture is necessary for purposeful movement'. The greater

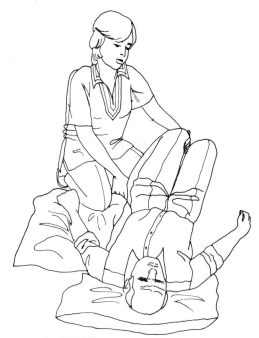

FIG. 42: HIP ROTATION, TO BE FOLLOWED BY BRIDGING.

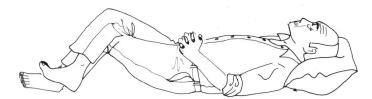

FIG. 43: RESTING WITHIN THE RECOVERY PATTERN.

part of hip rehabilitation takes place in routine rolling exercises. Bridging must be included and rolling must continue into rolling to sitting and rolling to crawling to high kneeling to knee walking to standing to walking. The exercises given here will be used in the proper time and place in the treatment programme to hasten recovery. The physiotherapist who is thoroughly experienced in stroke rehabilitation may use the sustained pressure splint to control overflow in the arm and to make use of finger-tip pressure while she works to facilitate controlled movement in the leg.

Figure 43, resting within the recovery pattern, shows a position some patients find very comfortable to adopt. The neck is slightly flexed, the arms rest comfortably with the handclasp maintaining an acceptable degree of external rotation of the shoulder, elbow extension and finger abduction. The affected leg is flexed and internally rotated at the hip and the sound leg is helping to maintain the correct position of the affected hip and giving pressure from the knee to the heel on the affected leg. If necessary, a pressure boot may be worn on the affected foot and the affected hip may be supported in flexion with internal rotation by a suitably placed sorbo rubber pad.

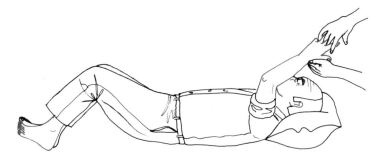

FIG.44: RECOVERY PATTERN ARM AND LEG.

Figure 44, recovery pattern arm and leg, demonstrates a handgrip which is frequently used to maintain finger and thumb abduction during shoulder rehabilitation. Consult Figure 7 for suitable handgrips. These handgrips are particularly important in all rehabilitation concerned with inhibiting the dominating reflexes and must be used to facilitate recovery where normal inhibiting influences are missing.

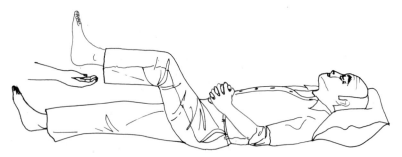

FIG.45: CONTROL OF THE AFFECTED LEG IN SPACE.

Figure 45, control of the affected leg in space, shows the patient who has re-established controlled hip movement, who has learnt to use active assisted movement to place the leg as in the diagram with the physiotherapist supporting his heel, who has felt approximation from knee to hip, who has learnt to control the knee in space (encouraged by brisk medial tapping on the knee joint if necessary), and who has finally achieved sustained posture in this position—or control of the leg in space—when the physiotherapist removes her hand from his heel.

These preliminary exercises have been illustrated to give an overall picture of the pattern rehabilitation takes. The intention is to demonstrate the following facts:

1. Diligent positioning continues during all treatment. At all times the body must be seen as a whole and positioned accordingly. If an exercise involves the upper extremity, the position of the lower extremity must be taken into account—and vice versa.

2. Redevelopment of normal movement is undertaken with the understanding that it is necessary to use the motor development patterns as seen in the infant to re-establish the postural reflex mechanism (with resulting normal muscle tone) and controlled movement.

3. Rolling over from supine uses the total flexion pattern and gives the first stage in our development pattern for our stroke patient. Almost all of the preliminary exercises are within this total flexion pattern.

4. Rolling over steps up sensory input, particularly to proprioceptors of muscle, stimulates tonic reflexes and postural mechanisms (e.g. the righting response) and, with the help of positioning, modifies the dominating reflexes.

5. Pressure splints are used to stimulate the spinal reflex arc (on which muscle tone is directly based) and at the same time, with correct positioning, to modify the dominating reflexes, to stabilise joints for early weight-bearing (approximation) and, where necessary, to boost sensory input to a high level by deep pressure.

6. The tonal pattern must be assessed frequently and techniques used to decrease or to increase muscle tone according to the findings. The tonal patterns can be expected to overlap and to co-exist.

7. Techniques used to decrease extensor muscle tone include positioning of limbs in total anti-spasm pattern, positioning and use of flexor dominant patterns as in roll over from supine, active assisted movement encouraging normal movement patterns with the physiotherapist maintaining the initiative and active assisted movement to place and hold limbs in space. Techniques used to increase extensor tone include deep pressure to stimulate the spinal reflex arc, approximation through joints with stability of deep pressure, approximation with weight transference and head extension to include the skilful use of tonic neck reflexes during arm rehabilitation.

8. As tonal patterns overlap, so do techniques. Where there is hypertonicity, extra care is taken to prevent drift into the tonic synergic pattern of rotation, to encourage normal movement patterns, and to mobilise into the anti-spasm pattern. Where there is hypotonicity, extra care is taken to stabilise the joints and mobilise into movement.

9. The direction of development of controlled movement is from

proximal to distal. Therefore, controlled movement in the hip and shoulder is established first. Development of movement over one joint will overlap with adjoining development.

10. The skill of the physiotherapist lies in her ability to understand the problems and principles of stroke treatment, to make accurate and reliable assessments and to tailor her treatment to fit the needs of each patient. The next stage in motor development involves rolling over to prone, prone-lying using the total extension pattern, and action must be taken to inhibit the dominating reflexes in the leg while making use of the extension pattern in arm rehabilitation.

Rolling from side to side in bed, rolling to sit on the edge of the bed, rising to standing and sitting beside the bed are all flexor dominated exercises. But activities in the prone position must be included in the planned use of the normal sequence of development of controlled movement for successful rehabilitation of the stroke patient. It is important to note at once that rolling to prone lying with forearm support *must* include the use of a pressure boot on the affected foot (or a square of sorbo rubber, or a pillow, to support the foot) to give mild flexion of the knee and to prevent full extension of the ankle *because rehabilitation has moved into the pattern of total extension.* Rolling to side-lying and maintaining side-lying is a total flexion pattern provided the patient is not trying to maintain balance against resistance towards the supine position. This means that any exercise given *against resistance* in the side-lying position will:

(a) produce the *flexion pattern* when the movement is towards the *prone position,* and

(b) produce the *extension pattern* when the movement is towards the *supine position.*

An extensor dominated exercise was used in rotation towards the supine position from side-lying in rehabilitation of shoulder and hip control. Prone lying with active extension of head and neck and forearm support is taught next. This brings in the symmetrical tonic neck reflex which increases extensor tone in the upper limbs. The prone position, and movement in the prone position—which includes crawling, knee walking and getting up to standing—must be used to lay the foundation for controlled walking. At the same time, the prone position must be used for successful arm rehabilitation. The skill of the physiotherapist lies in her ability to use this stage of rehabilitation to obtain maximum benefit, making full use of the tonic neck reflexes and at no time forgetting the need for careful positioning. The most frequent mistake that is made at this stage is neglect of correct leg positioning and not enough care is taken to prevent a build up of extensor tone in the lower limb. The shoulder is also frequently neglected. Internal rotation and a build up of extensor tone in the shoulder must not be allowed.

Correct positioning in prone lying with elbow support must include the following points (see Figs. 46 and 47).

(a) The forearms must be parallel, pointing straight forward to prevent internal rotation of the shoulder.

(b) The elbows must be directly below the shoulders, giving approximation from elbow to shoulder. The shoulders are stabilised in this position and approximation reinforced by manual pressure straight down through the shoulder.

(c) A pillow (or suitable padding) is placed low down under the shins to hold the ankles in good flexion and the knees in mild flexion. *Note* that reinforcement of gravity approximation by manual pressure is used repeatedly during the rehabilitation programme. In the forearm support position, if possible the fingers and thumb will be abducted. In the early days of treatment it is useful to instruct the patient frequently in the importance of thumb abduction so that the position becomes second nature to him—very soon he will usually be seen to use his sound hand to position the affected hand without being told. If the patient sags over to one side, resistance offered laterally to the opposite side will correct the position. When the patient has been thoroughly stabilised in this position, *prone-lying with forearm support,* transference of weight from side to side over alternate forearms is practised. With the approximation of the scapula to the head of the humerus, stretch is taken off the rotator cuff, shoulder stability is obtained and the painful shoulder syndrome is prevented.

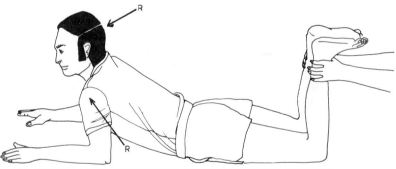

FIG. 46: PRONE-LYING WITH FOREARM SUPPORT, SHOULDERS STABILISED, ASSISTED KNEE FLEXION.

Figure 46 shows prone-lying with forearm support, shoulders stabilised and assisted knee flexion *in middle range.* This is a difficult exercise and is facilitated by using knees symmetrically. Vision will give a sensory boost if the long mirror is placed in front of the patient and he then controls and holds his neck position while he looks in the mirror to watch his legs. The tonic neck reflex helps to stabilise the arm position. The physiotherapist assists the leg movement, retaining the initiative and asking the patient to *think* about the movement... 'Think about the movement... We are going to bend and stretch your knees... Think about the movement... Feel the movement... Now help me to do it... *bend your knees* ...' It is essential to make every attempt to try and help the patient to retain the sensation of normal movement (here flexion and extension of the knees) in the brain's memory bank. Bilateral, or symmetrical, movement always helps here and is easier to perform than unilateral movement. This is an exercise which also assists in the maintenance of full hip extension. Rolling back into supine therapeutically is achieved by clasping the hands, palms touching and—turning the affected hand into supination—the patient is taught to press down with his sound hand and extend his sound elbow while he leads with his head turning towards the sound side and rolls, the body following the rotation of the head (the head righting reaction which leads to controlled rolling). He rolls over the affected side in an extensor dominated pattern. Again, proprioceptors on the affected side are stimulated by rolling. In a later progression he may extend his affected elbow and roll over the sound side.

Before he is taught to progress to movement, or crawling, in the prone position it is necessary for him to get up on to hands and knees—or into the crawling position—and to obtain stability in this position. Stability in the crawling position will be achieved fairly quickly if the patient is not pushed beyond his capabilities. His tolerance to exercise must always be considered and he must be treated accordingly. Each new position that is reached in his progression must be thoroughly stabilised before he is expected to move on.

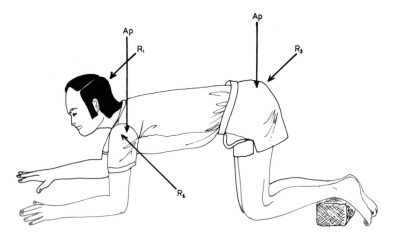

FIG.47: KNEELING WITH FOREARM SUPPORT, POSITION STABILISED.

Figure 47 shows kneeling with forearm support, position stabilised. The patient is balancing over his forearms. Initially the progression is achieved quite simply if the physiotherapist stands astride her patient, bends forwards to place her hands firmly round his iliac crests and lifts him upwards and backwards into the kneeling position. As far as he is able, he assists in the movement and draws his forearms backwards to achieve as nearly as possible 90° of flexion at his shoulders, elbows, hips and knees. At this stage in the rehabilitation programme he is usually quite ready to assist the change into the new position and he has enough shoulder control to draw the affected arm backwards into the required position. Resistance to the back of the head with upper cervical extension and lateral resistance to the affected shoulder again helps to stabilise the position. Resistance must be offered firmly and gently and built up slowly and withdrawn slowly. Remember that not until the patient maintains a steady position against reasonable resistance from *any* direction may he be said to be stabilised. It is necessary to emphasise that this method of stabilising adds strongly to the need for the maintenance of careful and correct positioning in the anti-spasm pattern so that firm resistance will not lead to build up of undesired spasticity. It is always necessary to consider whether an exercise is flexor dominated or extensor dominated and care must be taken to ensure that a correct demand is made to stimulate a desired (or correct) response. *Lateral stabilising* must not be forgotten. Transference of weight from side to side over alternate forearms is again practised. This is important because, apart from the necessary stimulus of approximation, rehabilitation is working on tonic reflexes—or reflexes which produce changes in muscle tone in relation to noxious stimuli and *weight transference.* Controlled weight bearing over the affected side must be established. While kneeling with forearm support, rocking backwards and forwards will also be practised. The wide base and low centre of gravity used in this exercise add a sense of security to the insecure patient. With fixed forearms (which are parallel, thumbs and fingers abducted) the patient learns to push backwards and forwards. *This is a treatment progression which must not be omitted.* The forearms must be used for support in prone with the forearms fixed and the trunk must be rocked over the forearms and hands to modify primitive movement patterns and *to re-educate controlled movement in the affected arm* just as the infant developed controlled movement. Later, in the crawling position, the patient will learn to balance over his hands. In the same way the primitive leg patterns are modified until controlled movement of hip and knee is developed.

It is always necessary to remember that exercise tolerance must be taken into account, that no two patients are the same and therefore the rehabilitation programmes must be tailored to suit individual requirements. The exercise sequence suggested here is simply an attempt to give a broad outline of treatment which includes:

(a) the necessary steps that must be taken if the stroke patient is to return to a full and normal life, and

(b) the stages in progress that lead to success.

Difficulties that present in any one patient must be faced and the physiotherapist must be prepared to look for ways and means of getting round problems so that the rehabilitation programme may continue and lead to success.

To give an example:

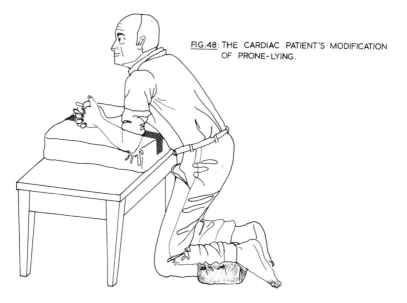

FIG.48: THE CARDIAC PATIENT'S MODIFICATION OF PRONE-LYING.

Figure 48 shows the cardiac patient's modification of prone lying. This diagram represents an elderly patient who came for physiotherapy treatment four months after onset of a dense left-sided hemiplegia. He lacked sitting and standing balance, had developed the typical marked spasm pattern on his left side and had considerable apraxic difficulties, particularly in dressing. He had had five previous incidents of myocardial infarct and a pace-maker had been inserted in his abdominal wall. He was unable to tolerate intensive exercise and this included prone lying. Figure 48 gives the modified position which he tolerated with ease and, in exercise sessions, he used it for increasing periods of time. He had contracted scar tissue from chest wall to the left shoulder which drew the shoulder into internal rotation and an old shoulder injury which added to the problem of correct shoulder positioning in external rotation. He also had an old fractured scaphoid which made supination of the hand with thumb abduction virtually impossible. As far as possible no stage in rehabilitation was left out. With good family support and an intensive course of treatment modified to suit his exercise tolerance and disabilities, he returned to an independent home life. This included toilet and dressing self-care and balanced walking with controlled and normal leg pattern, but, as might be expected, precision movements of the hand were not achieved. However, he had a painless shoulder with good scapula movement, arm elevation and controlled elbow movement.

Considering his disability and the initial four months of delay in starting treatment (he had not been correctly positioned during the initial four months after onset), this was a very fair degree of success, giving him an independent home life, and could in no way be classed as a failure. Early treatment would have achieved considerably more, as might continued intensive hospital rehabilitation. He had three months of intensive rehabilitation; thereafter, the value of continuing hospital treatment had to be weighed against the benefit to be gained by a return to home living as soon as possible. With his history, an early return to home life was obviously desirable and outweighed all other considerations.

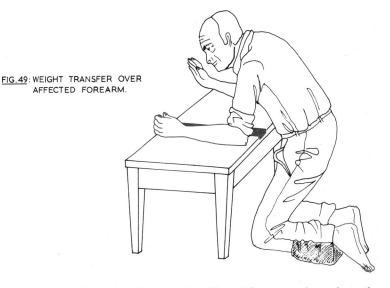

FIG.49: WEIGHT TRANSFER OVER AFFECTED FOREARM.

Figure 49, weight transfer over the affected forearm, shows how the same patient continued his rehabilitation programme. Note that it was not possible to spread his fingers and thumb into the anti-spasm pattern and he was concentrating on rotating the forearm into supination. Earlier in the programme a pressure splint had been used to facilitate shoulder movement; now it was found that a hand and wrist pressure splint facilitated hand positioning. This was used and tonic neck reflexes were brought into use to gain symmetrical and asymmetrical responses. Lateral transfers over the knees were practised, lateral shoulder resistance given gently to gain the required response to facilitate approximation over the affected forearm and gravity approximation was reinforced by manual pressure.

Figure 50, full kneeling with weight transfer over the affected side, is the next progression. The patient has now been weight-bearing from forearm to shoulder and from knee to hip, and this weight-bearing has been reinforced by manual pressure, but he has not been weight-bearing

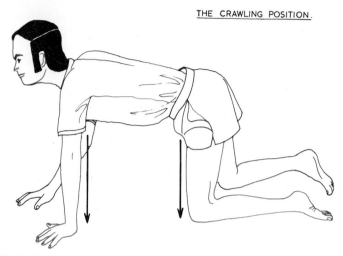

THE CRAWLING POSITION.

FIG. 50: FULL KNEELING, WEIGHT TRANSFER OVER AFFECTED SIDE,

from the proximal part of the palm of the hand to the shoulder. Arm rehabilitation depends on establishing this progression successfully. *Weight bearing from the heel of the hand through an extended elbow to a shoulder in external rotation is an essential step in rehabilitation if rehabilitation is to lead to recovery of precision movements of the hand.* To make this progression the patient must get up on to his hands in full kneeling (or the crawling position) as shown in Figure 50. At first it may be necessary for the physiotherapist to support the affected arm, holding the hand flat on the floor (fingers and thumb abducted) and the elbow

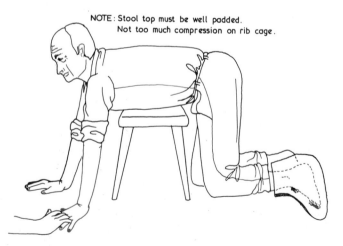

NOTE: Stool top must be well padded.
Not too much compression on rib cage.

FIG. 51: THE CARDIAC PATIENT'S AID TO FULL KNEELING, THE CRAWLING POSITION.

extended. She then removes the support she has given to her patient's hand and transfers her hand to give resistance to the back of his head with his neck in extension and lateral flexion to the affected side. This gains a response by stimulating the tonic neck reflex asymmetrically to give an increase in extensor tone in the affected arm. The fairly extreme degree of wrist extension necessary for this exercise is painless provided the pressure splint regime has been carefully followed. The increase in extensor tone in the arm facilitates triceps and the rehabilitation programme quickly reaches a point where manual support may be removed from the elbow. The patient is weight-bearing from the heel of his hand to his externally rotated shoulder. He is then thoroughly stabilised in this crawling position before crawling exercises are begun— and stabilising must include *lateral transfers* as in Figure 50. At this stage in treatment, support for the affected foot may usually be discontinued with no ill effects. If in *any doubt* about the need to continue diligent positioning to give the desired inhibiting influence on hypertonic motor neurones, then the affected foot should continue to be correctly supported or, a pressure boot will be worn for crawling exercises.

Up to this stage the rehabilitation programme has worked with the upper extremity, or with the lower extremity, but has not used alternating movements of arms and legs. The exercises given have been mainly symmetric. In rolling movement is one-sided, but controlled walking involves simultaneous movements asymmetrically of upper and lower extremities. To prepare for this, crawling exercises are used—as in infant development—but care should be taken to see that the exercise is not done as a haphazard routine.

Crawling: The patient is taught to move his limbs rhythmically as a continuation of proximal to distal development of controlled movement (Figure 50 continued). With the crawling position stabilised the patient is taught to rock backwards and forwards slowly. With resistance to backward rocking he pushes on his hands using arm extension, again with weight-bearing from the heel of the hand to the shoulder. Lateral rocking is also taught. It should be a slow, controlled movement and he is taught to hold his weight well over the affected side, balancing on the arm and leg from hand to shoulder and from hip to knee. Modified P.N.F. crawling exercises against resistance are very useful provided the physiotherapist understands positions for balance and total patterns of movement.

Positions for balance will be:

(a) Prone on forearms and knees—forearms parallel, knees and feet astride, feet more widely than knees.

(b) Prone on hands and knees, fingers and thumbs abducted with hands externally rotated, legs as above.

Total patterns of movement will be:

(a) Crawling on elbows and knees—forward and backward.

(b) Rocking on hands and knees—forward and backward.

(c) Crawling on hands and knees—forward and backward

The crawling progressions will be made at intervals in the rehabilitation programme when the patient is sufficiently stabilised and has gained the necessary proficiency to make a progression—and not before. The positions for balance maintain the necessary external rotation of the shoulder and internal rotation of the hip while the programme of weight-bearing (or approximation applied by gravity) is continued in all crawling exercise. Remembering that crawling forward is a flexor dominant pattern of movement and crawling backward is an extensor dominant pattern, the physiotherapist must use these exercises with skill, giving the correct manual resistance to achieve the required result. *With balancing in this crawling position on hands and knees and rocking backwards and forwards over the hands, the patient has begun the vital exercise to free the primitive flexor grasp and develop controlled hand movements.*

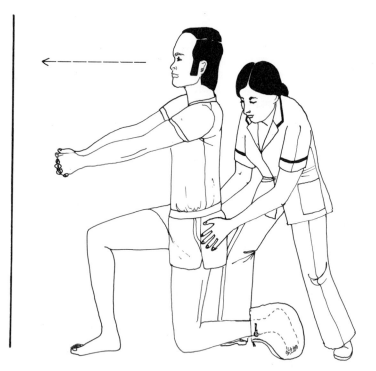

FIG. 52: STAND KNEELING (USING MIRROR) LEADING TO BALANCING OVER ALTERNATE KNEES AND PELVIC STABILISING WITH HIP CONTROL.

Figure 52: stand kneeling (using mirror) leading to balancing over alternate knees and stabilising with hip control, as might be expected, is a diagram which illustrates a whole series of progressions. It is the purpose of this book to set out a broad plan for physical rehabilitation of the stroke patient. Provided the important principles behind the plan are understood, and provided the plan is kept within the guide lines and uses the correct sequence for the development of controlled movement as seen in the infant, it may be suitably adapted and altered to suit the individual needs of each patient. But for all patients the correct sequence of development must be closely followed and correct positioning must be maintained. Where other physical complications make it difficult to follow all the progressions in rehabilitation as given here, modifications must be introduced so that the programme follows the guide lines set out as nearly as possible.

Kneeling—or stand kneeling—follows the crawling position. To get up into this position from prone kneeling the patient usually requires initial help. The physiotherapist may again stand astride her patient's legs and she flexes her own knees and ankles (as in the downhill skiing position) so that her knees prod his buttocks, giving sensory stimulation to assist his movement into the upright position. She leans forward, places her hands firmly on the anterior aspect of his shoulders, and assists him into the stand kneeling position. His hip extension may give a little initial difficulty. A few firm prods from the physiotherapist's knees will usually gain a satisfactory response. He *must* be stabilised in this position. It is a necessary step as the next progression in hip control—*but* it is much more than that, it is an essential step in the plan to establish effective cortical control. Here we are closely involved with *basal* level of reflex activity which gives us righting reflexes and equilibrium responses. In all rolling exercise the patient has been closely involved with the head righting reaction, now he moves into the upright position. The head righting reaction follows movement of the head in space with correction of eye level in response to disturbance of the labyrinth—the head rights, the body follows the head, leading to alignment of head, neck and trunk (this time vertically). The equilibrium response follows, tonic reflexes giving shifts in muscle tone with compensating movements to allow him to stand up to any altering situation caused by changes of position or environment. With stand kneeling, the patient depends on equilibrium responses to allow him to support his weight over this new fixed kneeling base and maintain balance. This is why he *must* be stabilised in this position. Equilibrium must be established. *Basal* responses are in part *cortical* and the physiotherapist must remember that *righting reflexes and equilibrium responses must be established before cortical level can be effective.* To assist in maintenance of the position a mirror is used to give a visual boost to sensory input. At first, the patient may be allowed to place his hands on a stool in front of him (hands correctly positioned, elbows extended) and to stabilise with arm support. Next he is taught to clasp his hands and lift them forwards off the stool as illustrated in Figure 52. Where it is necessary to step up sensory input the mirror is essential. If the floor mattress is made of thick sorbo rubber it assists development of equilibrium responses by giving a mildly unstable base, and positions the feet well if they are placed over the edge of the mattress. (Note that Figure 59 gives a very good modification of the high, or stand kneeling position.)

Manual pressure is used to teach the patient to hold the position, as in all stabilising of the rehabilitation positions, but as soon as the stand kneeling position has been thoroughly stabilised the patient is ready to begin the series of progressive exercises that follow. Manual pressure is now used to disturb the stable position and to obtain specific responses. Key points which control the strength and distribution of muscle tone in the rest of the body will be used and balance will be disturbed. The physiotherapist must remember that the greatest amount of movement (which always occurs when a patient holds against manual pressure) occurs at the greatest distance from the point used. For example, manual pressure against flexed fingers will gain a response in the feet if the resistance offered is maximal. The orthopaedic patient may be completely enclosed in plaster, but, if one of his great toes is free it can be used with maximal resistance to maintain muscle tone in the rest of the body. In stroke treatment, maximal resistance is the greatest amount of resistance which can be applied without defeating the purpose of the exercise and without producing unwanted activity in the hypertonic muscles. Where manual pressure is used to gain a response the same rule applies. Also, in the stroke patient's rehabilitation, when a position is stabilised and where manual pressure is used to disturb balance and gain a specific response, because we are redeveloping movement from proximal to distal, the choice of point of control will be central. The back of the head and pelvic and shoulder girdles are largely used. The thick sorbo rubber mattress will be sufficiently unstable to gain a response while, at the same time, it is sufficiently stable to eliminate the inhibiting reaction of fear. The desired response will not be obtained from a tense, frightened patient. He will simply respond to the stimulus of manual pressure by rigid loss of movement.

He is stabilised in the starting position, told to 'hold' the position, and the physiotherapist places her hands firmly in the correct position to gain a required response and pushes gently—or gives manual pressure— as she attempts to move him and he holds against her. The commands she gives must be short and easily understood . . . 'Hold . . . Stay where you are . . . Don't let me move you . . . Don't let me push you . . . Don't let me pull you . . .' Enough pressure must be given to gain the required response and time must be allowed to give a completed response. This means that the manual pressure, as always in stroke rehabilitation, is offered firmly and gently and built up slowly until the desired response is gained and then it is withdrawn slowly. Note that this is *not* the same technique as is used when prodding movements are given to gain a response. Prodding comes under the heading of brisk *tapping* which may be used as a sensory cue to prompt the patient to move a limb in a desired direction, or to gain a response by suddenly upsetting equilibrium. In the latter case it would be used at a later stage in the rehabilitation programme.

The rehabilitation programme has been working on gaining and strengthening controlled movement of hip and shoulder, on righting reactions, and is now particularly bringing in equilibrium responses. It has also reached the stage where exercise begins to concentrate on gaining and strengthening controlled movement of knee and elbow which is beginning to overlap with development of controlled movement in the foot and hand. *Strong manual pressure* will not cause harmful overflow, or irradiation, of muscle activity into synergic patterns of tonic contraction *if* it is used with skill and with expert and diligent use of correct positioning and movement into the recovery, or anti-spasm pattern. In other words, it should only be used with full understanding of the definition of maximal resistance as used in stroke rehabilitation, with intelligent use of the key points of tonic control (neck extension and trunk rotations), and therefore with full understanding of the problems involved. With understanding they cease to be problems, rehabilitation becomes a fascinating, worthwhile and rewarding exercise and the patient's future outlook is bright. Dominant reflexes will be inhibited, hypertonicity will not be allowed to develop into marked muscle spasm, neither will it be forgotten that hypotonicity is also a problem and weak muscles must be strengthened. The skill of the physiotherapist lies in her ability to identify the abnormal tonal patterns, to plan and carry out a correct and dynamic rehabilitation programme, and to re-educate to normal.

To give an obvious example of one use of manual pressure facilitating recovery in the stroke patient when stand kneeling has been established, manual pressure to the posterior chest wall will stimulate postural reflexes and equilibrium responses (by disturbing balance) and *initiate contraction of the hamstrings.* Holding of symmetrical and asymmetrical neck extension will be used and holding against trunk rotations. Lateral transference of weight must be carefully taught. Trunk rotations lead on to weight transference, lateral transfers obviously include counter rotation of pelvis and shoulders. The physiotherapist ought to work out the sequence of movement on her own body if she is in any doubt about the movement she is asking her patient to make. If she herself goes down into stand kneeling and transfers her weight correctly over one hip and knee she will feel the counter rotation of her shoulders on her pelvis.

The patient is in stand kneeling with his knees astride and lower legs parallel and he is taught to transfer his weight over one hip and knee. His stance must be erect. Again the stool may be brought into use to advantage if he places his hands, correctly positioned, on the top of the stool and supports himself with extended elbows on externally rotated shoulders. Tonic neck reflexes will be used to stabilise the position and manual approximation down through the shoulders may also be given. With this position established the patient will be taught to transfer his weight over one hip and knee and one hand and then to develop a stable and rhythmical slow movement from side to side, balancing over controlled shoulder and hip joints. If this exercise gives any difficulty, it should be facilitated if the physiotherapist gives manual pressure straight down through both shoulders, or from the brim of the pelvis down through the hips (but the hips must not be flexed), or she may simply stabilise the affected elbow with one hand while she uses her other hand to give manual pressure down through the affected shoulder. If necessary, prodding over the gluteal region will assist hip extension. Remember also, if there is still difficulty in establishing the stand kneeling position, *basal* responses include the head righting reaction. If the physiotherapist places her fingers under her patient's chin and lifts his head, head and neck will move into correct alignment and lumbar extension follows.

In stand kneeling where the stool is not used, the patient will clasp his hands (palms touching, elbows extended) to practise lateral transference of weight. The physiotherapist will kneel behind him, and, placing her hands on the brim of his pelvis, she will again give manual pressure downwards before she gives gentle pressure to assist his rhythmical slow movement from side to side. *She will direct the movement laterally and forwards over the affected hip* and she will continue to give this manual direction into the correct hip weight-bearing pattern until he joins in the movement and controlled movement takes over.

Step by step, all through the beginning series of exercises, the aim has been to establish normal upright posture over a controlled hip. Beginning with bridging, exercises have been working steadily towards this end. *Normal upright posture over a controlled hip* **must** *be established* before normal controlled walking can be expected. If the patient fails to weight-bear in stand kneeling over a controlled hip as described above the physiotherapist must consider she has failed to reach her objective and, before she proceeds with her treatment programme, she must go back to the beginning and concentrate on bridging. Bridging may be used bilaterally or unilaterally against resistance, followed by hip rotations, rolling and resisted crawling (care being taken to make sure that hip extension is not lost) and the exercises will be repeated over and over again until the necessary goal is reached. Modified bridging with the sound leg in extension and the affected leg crossed over the sound leg in the crook position can be a useful exercise position. Resistance is used against the affected knee to raise the affected buttock and start hip rotation while maintaining hip protraction. Where treatment is not undertaken and properly established in the early days, the patient's whole rehabilitation is put at risk—which leads me to insist that stroke treatment must be *early*, intensive and of sufficient duration to gain the required response.

The physiotherapist will remember to use the techniques necessary to decrease muscle tone where necessary. In this case, as well as maintaining careful positioning for all exercise, *active assisted* movements will be used, the physiotherapist maintaining the initiative so that excessive effort will not lead to *unwanted irradiation and stimulation (instead of inhibition) of dominant reflexes.*

Controlled walking may be preceded by controlled knee walking. The physiotherapist kneels beside her patient *on his affected side* and holds his affected arm as in Figure 7g—arm in external rotation, elbow extended, wrist extended and thumb abducted—and, with lateral transference of weight over the affected side, weight is distributed through the affected shoulder to the heel of the hand and through the affected hip and knee, freeing the sound hip and knee to take a step. With this routine carefully established, knee walking with correct transference of weight is begun and the patient and the physiotherapist knee walk side by side, practising until the movement becomes easy routine. The patient may then clasp his hands, palms touching, elbows extended, and begin knee walking alone, an exercise which should be carefully and thoroughly mastered because of its importance in the scheme to train symmetrical control of a whole body. In this position with correct lateral transference of weight, the patient is using his affected hip in the normal pattern for controlled walking without allowing any chance of movement into the extensor spasm pattern. He is, in fact, performing formal balanced walking with weight transference over the affected side. The patient who has not mastered lateral transference of weight over the affected hip will be found to hold his weight over the sound hip with a sagging pelvis while he attempts to move the affected leg forward on a flexed hip—which is usually adducted and internally rotated—with a flexed lumbar spine. In this case, not surprisingly, the patient is in trouble and it is easy to understand why it is necessary to take great care with lateral stabilising.

The other consideration which must not be forgotten is the therapeutic value of self-care exercise and the cheerful optimism the average patient will attain when he is successfully led forward by a series of useful self-care exercises which he knows are giving daily physical improvement and leading to a return to independence. At this stage the patient can often be trusted to carry out a series of mat exercises alone—or with minimal supervision—without perpetuating bad habits with trick movements and bad positioning. Such a self-care programme will be of tremendous value both mentally and physically and will include exercises in rolling, bridging, hip and shoulder rotations, rolling to elbow propping, prone lying with forearm support, crawling and kneeling. If he has been carefully and repeatedly instructed in correct positioning and working into the recovery pattern from the beginning, he will usually automatically stay out of the spasm pattern. Exercises which follow motor development of the infant using mainly free mass flexion patterns, and the method described here using hand-clasps to maintain the arm recovery pattern, will not lead to unwanted irradiation and resulting excessive reflex dominant tone.

In rolling it must be remembered that the eyes lead the movement, followed by turning of the head, followed by simultaneous rotation of the shoulders and arm movement—hands clasped with arms in elevation. Several patients may be treated together, provided there is a very large floor mat and one physiotherapist to supervise. Group therapy has a very beneficial effect. The cheerful, go-ahead patient will encourage his slower companions and competition in progress will result. One patient's correction of another's faulty position often has greater impact than correction from the physiotherapist. Repeated rolling, *correctly carried out* with several revolutions in quick succession and practised in both directions facilitates crawling balance particularly where extensor spasm of the leg is threatening to give trouble. The reason for this ought by now to be thoroughly understood—trunk rotation inhibiting spasm and rolling stimulating head righting.

Note: all resting periods during mat work ought to be given with the patient in side-lying with correct positioning. Supine lying and the consequent build up of extensor spasm must be avoided. It is important to continue with the rigid programme necessary to inhibit the dominating reflexes. Counter rotation of pelvis and shoulders must be included because of this need and may be practised in the group activity class in crook lying, head, shoulders and arms rotating to one side while knees are rotated to the opposite side. Lying on the affected side must be included, particularly where there is sensory loss, to give pressure stimulation and hip extension (with the knee flexed) as in Figure 25.

Where elbow extension is not yet suitably stable to carry out crawling exercise on all fours, crawling on forearms (Fig. 47) will be used in the group class. Measures must be taken to stimulate joint proprioceptors and postural reflexes in the arm. Where several patients need assistance with elbow support, forearm crawling would be used while assistance with elbow support must be given individually, with extra assistance outwith the class. This assistance must include:

1. Use of the pressure splint—with intermittent pressure where proprioceptive sense is seriously impaired.

2. Use of the pressure splint—with sustained pressure given by the orally inflated splint.

3. Constant repetition of the series of pressure splint exercises (using the orally inflated splint) taking particular care to practise *approximation* from the heel of the hand to a protracted shoulder in external rotation (see Fig. 34). This last exercise is of the utmost importance and,

where possible, an assistant should be asked to support the shoulder firmly in protraction and give the necessary counter-pressure. I am convinced that this exercise is an essential part of all successful arm rehabilitation and also offers the solution to the vexed, long standing problem of residual disability because of sensory loss. In this case it *must* be part of the intensive treatment programme and *must* be included in every treatment session. If there is not sufficient time for the individual's planned programme to be undertaken on any one day, or if his exercise tolerance proves to be lower on any one day, whatever else is omitted, this *arm approximation under pressure ought not to be omitted*

In this last series of exercises the patient has now reached the stage where he should be ready to practise the exercise as shown in Figure 52.

Figure 52, balancing over alternate knees and pelvic stabilising with hip control, illustrates the next progression. The patient's head is correctly positioned (with mirror aid), his lumbar spine is extended, his weight has been transferred laterally over the affected hip giving weight bearing on the knee with forward rotation of the pelvis (encouraged by manual pressure) and the sound leg has been lifted forward with the foot correctly positioned. Again, if there is initial difficulty in establishing the position, the physiotherapist may kneel on her patient's affected side and encourage lateral transference of weight by using the arm grip as in Figure 7g. But, where kneeling balance and knee walking have been properly undertaken, this new position is usually easily achieved. Control over the affected hip in this new position must be established. Central manual pressure is used with both hands placed with thumbs along the brim of the pelvis; also brisk tapping (I prefer the word 'prodding' which suggests firm tapping with rigid fingers) over the affected buttock, and trunk rotation, head, neck, shoulders and arms moving over a fixed pelvis.

The sound leg is placed back into the kneeling position, the weight is transferred over the sound hip and the affected leg is lifted forward on to the foot. It is not suitable to practise this exercise with a pressure boot on. I prefer the use of a thick floor mat with the patient kneeling with his feet over the edge of the mat. As in the whole rehabilitation programme, limb positioning is all important and the patient may need help with the affected foot when he lifts it forward. It must be placed so that approximation by gravity takes place from the knee to the heel and this approximation will be reinforced by manual pressure. The patient will be taught to hold the knee at a right angle in the mid-position. If the hip drifts into external rotation, brisk tapping on the inner aspect of the knee will bring it back into position.

With the full establishment of this series of exercises in stand kneeling the patient is ready to get up off the floor unaided. The physiotherapist must make sure that he is thoroughly stabilised in all the required positions. If not, she will assess his difficulty carefully and deal with it.

Figure 53, lateral transfer in kneeling, shows another method that may be used to obtain the desired result. It can be a useful hold for an elderly patient who has initial difficulty in establishing stand kneeling balance and needs the added security of additional support from his physiotherapist to inhibit the fear that comes with holding his head high in space. His arm is well positioned with a protracted and externally rotated shoulder and the physiotherapist has a free hand to assist in hip control with the manual pressure necessary to encourage lateral weight transfer. The pressure should be offered gently and firmly, pulling the pelvis forwards into protraction before pushing gently laterally towards the sound side.

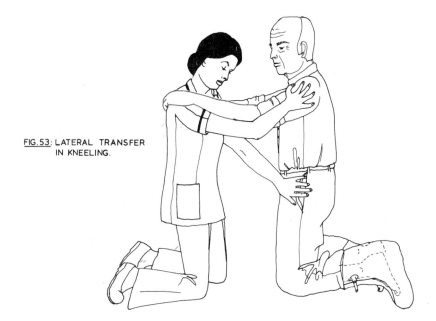

FIG.53: LATERAL TRANSFER IN KNEELING.

Figure 54, lateral transfer over affected hand (using two stools), again gives the nervous patient an additional feeling of security in an essential exercise which he can practise by himself provided he is correctly positioned and stabilised. The affected knee must not be allowed to drift out of position. Cross facilitation may be used here to advantage. The patient will be taught to transfer his weight forwards over his affected foot and lift his sound hand and carry it across to place it beside his affected hand. Assistance with elbow support may be necessary and added help will be given by using asymmetrical neck extension to the affected side against resistance. Again, the position of the affected foot is very important. The heel must be firmly on the floor so that the body weight is transferred over the heel to give the normal weight bearing

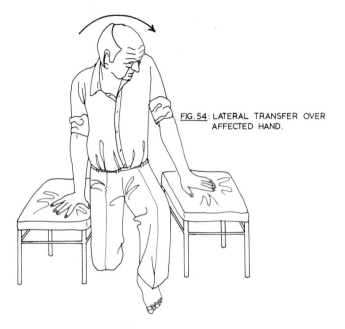

FIG.54: LATERAL TRANSFER OVER
AFFECTED HAND.

position of the foot. Where a tendency towards developing spasm is a
problem, the spasm pattern may be further reduced by separating the
toes with small pieces of sponge-rubber.

Figure 55a, b, getting up from the floor on to a stool, is easily
accomplished if the treatment programme has followed the lines set
down above. From the stand kneeling position alongside the stool, the
patient places his sound hand firmly on the stool, lifts his sound leg
forwards to place the foot firmly on the floor, and, leaning forwards, he
pushes on the hand and foot, raises his buttocks and pivots round into a
sitting position. The diagram is self-explanatory.

Stool exercises

The stool is an essential aid to successful stroke rehabilitation. It
should be of a suitable height for the patient to sit with his hips, knees
and ankles flexed to 90°, wide enough to support the buttocks and
thighs, and long enough to support both hands with the arms held in
good abduction. The starting position for all stool exercises must be
correct—*the shoulder must not be allowed to turn into internal rotation
or the hip into external rotation.* The following points should be noted:

1. The patient may sit with both arms extended in external rotation at
the shoulders, elbows extended and palms placed flat on the top of the
stool with fingers and thumbs abducted.

2. The patient may sit with his affected arm in the above position (1)
while he carries out exercises in cross facilitation with the sound arm.

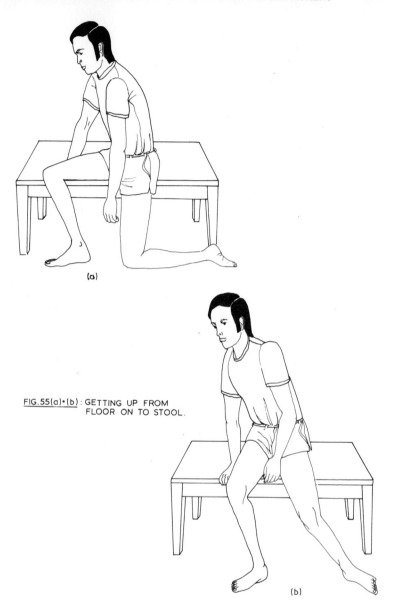

(a)

FIG.55(a)·(b) : GETTING UP FROM
FLOOR ON TO STOOL.

(b)

3. The patient may sit with his hands clasped in front, fingers interlaced, palms touching and elbows extended.

4. The patient may sit in the above position (3) and then flex his elbows to place them firmly on his knees and lean in this position (giving approximation of knee to heel and shoulder to elbow). This ensures

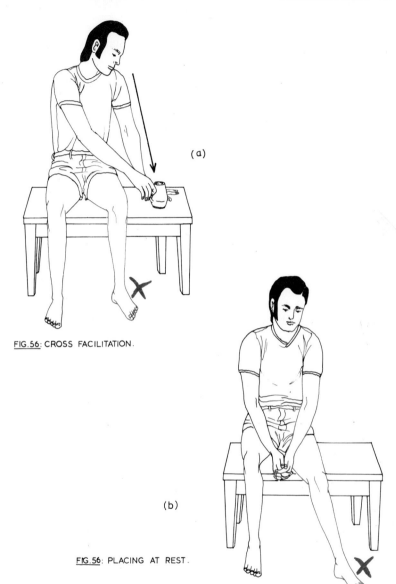

FIG.56: CROSS FACILITATION.

(a)

(b)

FIG.56: PLACING AT REST.

good shoulder positioning for all stool exercise. Hip positioning is equally important and the following point must be noted:

5. In all four of the above positions the patient must sit with his knees parted and flexed to 90° with his heels directly below his knees. The following list of exercises gives a suggested outline for rehabilitation

using the stool but, by now, it will be understood that the physiotherapist is assessing her patient very carefully and planning his exercise routines according to the disability she finds.

Exercise 1: stabilising sitting balance. Balance has been thoroughly stabilised, or training has been undertaken, in the crawling and kneeling positions, and it ought to be thoroughly stabilised in sitting before walking re-education begins. Sitting correctly positioned on the stool—with no back support to encourage leaning backward and slumping on the seat—makes an immediate demand on the patient and gains a response. He maintains his upright position. This is routine physiotherapy and, if the necessary preliminary exercises have been given, it should pose no problems here. For stabilising exercises, the important point to remember is that *the starting position must be correct.* The patient is taught to sit upright with knees astride, feet immediately below the knees, and hips, knees and ankles flexed to 90°. He clasps his hands in front, elbows extended, and is stabilised in this position.

Exercise 2: leaning backward on extended elbows. The patient sits with both arms extended in external rotation at the shoulders, elbows extended and palms placed flat on top of the stool with fingers and thumbs abducted. Care should be taken to position the feet correctly. Initially the physiotherapist will give support to the affected elbow while she works on the tonic neck reflexes to increase extensor tone in the arm. She gives manual resistance symmetrically to neck extension and, at the same time, withdraws (or lessens) her support to the affected elbow. When necessary she will increase extensor tone still further in the affected arm by giving asymmetrical neck extension against resistance to the affected side. *Note:* she must watch the leg position carefully.

Exercise 3: cross facilitation (see Fig. 56a). The first point to note is that the affected foot has not been correctly positioned—or enough care has not been taken to ensure that total correct positioning is maintained throughout all exercise. As shown in the diagram, the affected leg has been allowed to drift towards the spasm pattern—hip rolling slightly into external rotation and foot into plantar flexion. Compare the position with the position of the sound leg. The drift towards the spasm pattern has been illustrated here to pinpoint the need to see the body as a whole and to pay constant attention to correct positioning, not forgetting the lower limb while working with the upper limb, and vice versa. Note that the stool gives a suitable base to allow full rotation over the affected arm. The exercise involves weight transfer over the hand, hip and foot—emphasising the need for diligent care in positioning. *Weight must always be transmitted through a correctly positioned base.* No opportunity of putting this valuable principle of cross facilitation into practice should be neglected (that is, using the sound side of the body across midline to initiate bilateral activity). Figure 56a illustrates the coffee break; it also illustrates the need for constant supervision of positioning. If the patient had not succeeded in weight-bearing over an extended elbow at this stage, his coffee would have been placed on a higher table on his left-hand side so that he lifted his head as he rotated to reach for the cup—neck extension is often all that is needed to facilitate the exercise.

Exercise 4: sitting with palms placed sideways on the top of the stool, shoulders in external rotation with elbows extended, weight transfer to cross one leg over the other. Practise alternate leg crossing.

Exercise 5: sitting with hands clasped, legs correctly positioned, elbows flexed and placed firmly on the knees, leaning forward to give approximation of shoulder to elbow and knee to heel.

Exercise 6: sitting with hands clasped, legs correctly positioned, elbows extended, leaning forward to touch the floor with the knuckles— weight is transferred forward over the hips to the thighs and down through the heels. Change the starting position to sitting with knees and feet together and practise leaning forward to touch the floor on alternate sides of the legs.

Exercise 7: sitting with hands clasped, elbows extended, cross one leg over the other and rotate the head, shoulders and extended arms to the opposite side (counter rotation of shoulders and pelvis). Practise alternate leg crossing with counter rotation (extensor spasm inhibiting pattern).

Exercise 8: haunch walking with hands clasped, elbows extended. This movement involves weight transfer from hip to hip, the transfer of weight freeing the non weight-bearing hip which is lifted clear of the stool and moved forward one small step. There is room on the stool for four steps forward and four back.

Exercise 9: sitting with palms placed sideways on top of the stool, shoulders in external rotation, weight transfer over the hands and feet to lift the buttocks clear of the stool. As soon as this exercise is mastered it may be done with lateral movement, lifting the buttocks from side to side.

Exercise 10: sitting on the stool (Fig. 56b), placing the leg in space and holding it there. As illustrated, the patient has not maintained the 'placed' position because of dominating reflexes and the leg has drifted into external rotation and dropped slowly to the floor. Where this happens it is necessary to go back in the treatment programme and check all positioning in every situation with very great care and continue with assisted movement. The ability to maintain a limb in space is lost to the stroke patient because of changes in muscle tone. As rehabilitation progresses and normal tone is restored the 'placing' ability is also restored. If the foot position is not maintained correctly by the patient in Exercise 3 he will not be ready to begin Exercise 10.

Exercise 11: standing up and sitting down. Figure 57 gives some helpful suggestions where difficulty is encountered in establishing this exercise. Here again, the physiotherapist is using her knees to support her patient's knees, leaving her hands free to control his pelvic move-

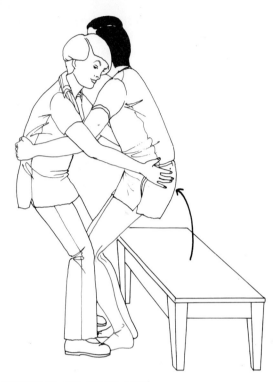

FIG.57: STANDING UP AND SITTING DOWN.

1st .COMMAND: "Lean well forward .... and stand up!"
The physiotherapist's body prevents the patient's affected arm from falling into the pattern of spasm, her arm grips and controls his elbow, her hand controls his hip, her knees control his knees.

2nd .COMMAND: "Lean well forward .... and sit down!"

NOTE : Sitting balance must be thoroughly established on the stool. Haunch walking forwards , backwards and laterally should also be practised.

ment so as to encourage weight transference forward over the apex of the longtitudinal arches of his feet, and her arm grips and supports his affected arm in a good position. The aim is for the patient to stand up from the stool unassisted with his hands clasped and elbows extended. He reaches his hands forward and leans to transfer his weight over his feet and lifts his buttocks clear of the stool (as in Exercise 9 minus hand support). This may be practised as a rocking movement and, as confidence is gained and postural reactions facilitated in the affected leg, standing will follow. At this stage, to establish the exercise, supporting assistance may be given in the following two ways:

(a) The physiotherapist may grasp her patient's clasped hands *provided he does* **not** *pull to standing.* He is learning to transfer weight correctly so that the line of gravity falls through his instep. To do this, *he must push* forward to standing.

(b) As soon as he pushes forward to transfer his weight over his feet, the physiotherapist may transfer one of her hands to the back of his head to give mild resistance to neck extension accompanied by an upward thrust—but this second use of supporting assistance should not be offered until his buttocks are clear of the stool.

Exercise 12: Figure 58 shows the position for lateral stabilising using the stool. Lateral stabilising is of the utmost importance and no rehabilitation programme must neglect this vital step in the treatment programme. It is a help if each exercise in lateral stabilising in sitting is

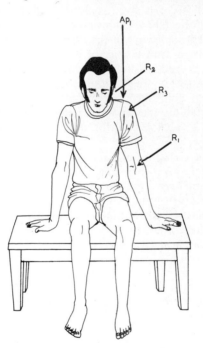

FIG.58: LATERAL STABILISING.

1) $\underline{Ap_1 + R_1}$: Ap_1, or Approximation, from shoulder to hand with R_1, or Resistance, to stabilise the elbow

2) $\underline{R_2 + R_1}$: R_2, or Resistance to the back of the head to give spinal extension and facilitate extensor pattern, or thrust, in the arms.

3) $\underline{R_3}$: R_3, or Resistance laterally at the shoulder will finally maintain position.

preceded by a short session of shoulder to hand approximation, supporting assistance being given to the affected elbow where necessary. Postural reactions must be stimulated in the affected arm at every opportunity to facilitate successful treatment. As illustrated in Figure 58, the following routine has been undertaken.

(a) Gravity approximation from the shoulder to the hand was reinforced by manual pressure down through the shoulder with supporting assistance to maintain elbow extension.

(b) The patient transferred his weight over his affected hand and a mild degree of elbow flexion was allowed. He was taught to push on his hand and to extend the elbow with assistance, to extend the elbow without assistance, and finally to extend the elbow against R_1—or gentle resistance offered against extension.

(c) Resistance (R_2) was given asymmetrically to neck extension with rotation to reinforce elbow extension against R_1.

(d) Lateral Resistance at the shoulder—R_3—was given to promote and maintain lateral transference of weight over the affected side.

This suggested series of stool exercises will lead to full stability in sitting, re-education of weight transference over the affected side in sitting, increased controlled hip movement, stimulation of postural reactions and stability in standing up from sitting while, at the same time, they make a valuable contribution towards successful arm rehabilitation.

Exercises which lead to full stability in standing—with lateral transference of weight over the affected leg and walking over a fully controlled hip and knee—must now be included in the treatment plan. It is proposed here to continue with a series of suggested exercises (and exercise positions) which will meet our purpose and also successfully cope with any difficulties that may be encountered. It will be noted that at no time is the arm forgotten and that arm and leg rehabilitation proceed simultaneously.

As soon as the patient has learnt to stand up, the physiotherapist must make sure he knows the correct and safe way to approach a chair and sit down on it. This means that the suitably broad based chair—with solid forearm rests and comfortably upright back—is placed in front of him while he is sitting on the stool. He leans forward to place his hands on the seat of the chair. Hands and feet must be correctly positioned. He is taught to lean on his hands and stand up while the physiotherapist continues to give supporting assistance to the affected elbow where necessary. He may stand in this position, weight-bearing on all four limbs, to advantage. It makes an excellent starting position for further four limb weight-bearing exercises and approximation with manual pressure, stabilising and lateral transfers should all be used. Next he stands upright facing the chair and bends forward to place his hands on the arm rests, or the physiotherapist will support the affected arm as in Figure 7g, and, with balance safely established in this position, he lifts his sound hand and transfers it across to the other arm rest and turns slowly towards the sound side to sit down. As soon as this manoeuvre is safely established, it must be impressed on the patient that at any time he approaches a chair he must walk right up to it before he leans to place his sound hand firmly on the arm rest. Drill in transferring the sound hand from one arm rest across to the other and turning to sit on the chair ought to begin at an early stage in treatment, therefore it is most likely the physiotherapist will be using the handgrip as in Figure 7g.

Parallel bars

The patient is now ready to begin work in the parallel bars—*but he is not yet ready to begin walking in the parallel bars.* Lateral transfer of weight over the affected hip in standing must be established first. The necessary equipment for this stage in rehabilitation will include parallel bars, two suitable chairs, a stool and a full-length mirror on wheels. *The mirror is essential,* particularly where sensory loss is involved. *The parallel bars ought not to be used as a means of pulling to standing* with the sound arm, *or as a means of maintaining balance by supporting on the sound side.* Almost without exception, every approach that is made to the patient and all assistance offered is from the affected side, and successful rehabilitation depends on this method of approach. To allow the patient to depend on his unaffected side for support is to move into the danger area of compensating for disability with the sound side and, if this is allowed, it will spoil the treatment plan and ruin the programme that is leading the patient back to normal living. To compensate for disability with the sound side is to actively prevent recovery of the affected side. Therefore, the parallel bars must not be used by the sound side to compensate for the disabled side. Using the parallel bars wrongly in this way is one of the commonest mistakes made in well-meaning but disastrous treatment programmes. This is why I would say 'the patient is not yet ready to begin walking in the parallel bars'. *Lateral balance over the affected side in standing must be established first.*

Having reached an erect posture standing in the parallel bars, standing balance is essential to maintain this posture. If the patient achieved the exercises illustrated in Figure 52, this next advance in his training will not be difficult. Maintenance of correct erect posture is dependent on postural responses and the whole programme of rehabilitation has been directed towards this end. For *maintenance of correct posture* study the following notes.

Note on the ankle and foot: The patient must stand on a correctly positioned foot. This means that *weight must be transmitted through the heel* with the whole of the foot resting on the floor. If he is to stand properly, the patient's standing base must be correct. If necessary the foot will be placed in position by the physiotherapist. *The ankle must not be held in plantar flexion with the heel off the floor and the forefoot resting on the metatarsal heads.* With the heel correctly placed, postural reactions in the leg will again be given a boost by applying manual pressure downwards from hips to heels. The physiotherapist places her hands on the patient's iliac crests with firm manual contact and applies strong pressure downwards in vigorous thrusts.

Note on the pelvis and lumbar spine: The patient lifts his head and examines his standing position in the mirror. Body alignment follows the head movement and neck extension stimulates tonic neck reflexes, increasing extensor tone in the upper limbs and trunk to assist in establishing the upright position. This means that provided the head is correctly positioned the pelvis will rotate forwards and the lumbar spine will extend.

Note on arm position: The patient may keep his hands resting on the parallel bars which are then adjusted to the correct height to give weight transfer from the heel of the hand to the shoulder through an extended elbow. With the arms in mild abduction and the hands in front of the body, the shoulders will be well positioned in external rotation with protraction.

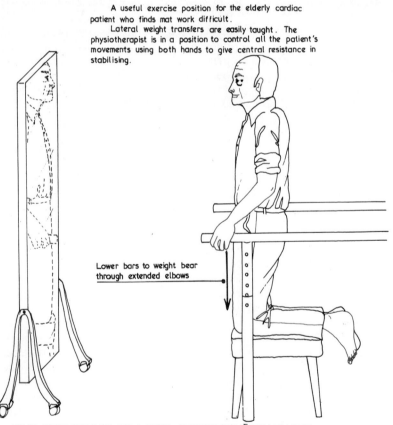

A useful exercise position for the elderly cardiac patient who finds mat work difficult.

Lateral weight transfers are easily taught. The physiotherapist is in a position to control all the patient's movements using both hands to give central resistance in stabilising.

Lower bars to weight bear through extended elbows

FIG.59: STAND KNEELING ON A STOOL BETWEEN THE PARALLEL BARS.

Figure 59 gives an exercise position that can be very useful, particularly where the whole sequence of exercise as given for Figure 52 was not mastered Weight transfer over the affected hip in stand kneeling ought to be mastered before it is taught in standing. A stool with a thick, soft, padded top will stimulate equilibrium responses as well as being comfortable for the knees. To get up into the kneeling position on the stool, the patient transfers his weight over the affected leg and lifts the sound knee up on to the stool. If this movement presents any problems, the physiotherapist will use both of her hands to give pelvic supporting control and to assist in lateral transfer of weight over the affected hip, freeing the sound knee which is lifted forward on to the stool. He then stands on the sound knee and brings the affected leg up into position so that he is kneeling as in Figure 59. Or, it may still be necessary for her to support the affected elbow with one hand while she uses her other hand to assist in pelvic control. In both cases, therefore, she obviously takes up her own position standing behind her patient. He is taught to hold this position with his knees slightly astride and his lower legs parallel. Using the mirror, he corrects his own head position and his body comes into alignment in an erect posture. If he does not like the feeling of space in front of him and lacks security, a high-backed chair may be placed in front of the stool with its back towards him. It will give him confidence and remove his fear of falling forward, but, for obvious reasons, it must not obstruct his mirror image of his head and shoulders.

The physiotherapist steps forward to stand between her patient's feet, leaving the feet free over the edge of the stool. This controls the position of his lower leg—and therefore the position of his hip—and leaves both of her hands free to control his posture centrally from pelvic level. This places her in an ideal situation to assist his pelvic control and is particularly useful when he has lost awareness of his pelvic position.

Note: If the earlier stages in rehabilitation of hip control have not been followed, it is frequently found that the stroke patient weight-bears on the sound side with a pelvic sag to the same side accompanied by flexion in the lumbar spine. These postural symptoms indicate neglect of correct rehabilitation procedures in the early days and—because of the lapse of time—they are not easy to deal with. Where this has occurred it is often necessary to go right back to the beginning, especially making sure that bridging is established, and stand kneeling as illustrated here will be used intensively in the rehabilitation programme. The exercises which may be taught include:

Exercise 1: kneeling balance.

Exercise 2: lateral transfer of weight over affected knee and hand.

Exercise 3: knee walking—two small steps backward and two forward.

Exercise 4: approximation from shoulder to knee through a controlled hip, or from pelvis to knee, with manual pressure.

Exercise 5: approximation from shoulder to the heel of the hand through an extended elbow (with parallel bars adjusted to the suitable height and, where necessary, assistance with elbow support).

Exercise 6: bilateral weight transfers over controlled hips with hands clasped in elevation.

Exercise 7: kneeling with hands clasped in elevation, shoulder rotation over the pelvis.

If maintenance of hip position gives trouble and the patient sags into flexion, the physiotherapist will give prodding over the buttocks using rigid fingers to act as a sensory reminder. Then, for correct lateral transfer of weight over the hip, she may again find it necessary to place her hands on the brim of his pelvis and assist his movement laterally and forwards *over* the hip. The exercise must remain in the treatment programme and continue to be practised with care until the patient can maintain good hip control independently.

Exercises in the parallel bars in standing

The physiotherapist continues to take up her position behind her patient and she will stand, or sit on a stool, depending on the control point she is using. The patient's foot must be very carefully positioned for all standing and walking exercise (refer to note above) so that weight is transmitted through the heel. If the foot is not positioned correctly the leg will not be used correctly and the rehabilitation plan will fail. If necessary, help will be given to position the foot. As the patient moves his weight over the foot, help will also be given to:

(a) maintain correct limb posture and

(b) reinforce postural reflexes.

(a) *To maintain correct limb posture,* the physiotherapist will use manual pressure to assist her patient to transfer his weight laterally and forwards over the hip. She may also use her knee to give supporting assistance to his knee to prevent hyperextension and to assist in knee stabilising.

(b) *To reinforce postural reflexes,* she will use manual pressure to increase gravity approximation from hip to heel through a controlled knee—as above.

Some physiotherapists prefer to do these standing exercises at the wallbars but, if the patient stands inside the parallel bars, he is in a suitable position to practise approximation from hand to shoulder and the position of the bar assists in maintenance of the necessary external rotation of the affected shoulder for all of the exercises.

Exercise 1: standing, stabilising.

Exercise 2: approximation. The physiotherapist takes up her position standing behind her patient. He stands with his legs slightly astride and, if necessary, she will give help in placing his affected foot correctly. The bars are adjusted to allow his hands to hold a weight-bearing position with extended elbows. Using the mirror he corrects his own head position. Approximation is applied by the physiotherapist with manual pressure from the brim of the pelvis down to the heel. Retraction of the pelvis is not allowed and supporting assistance will be given to the knee if necessary (as above). Approximation is also applied from the shoulder to the heel of the hand through an extended elbow. Again supporting assistance will be given to the elbow if necessary.

Exercise 3: weight transfer over the affected hip. The correct foot position must be maintained, retraction of the pelvis must not be allowed, and the patient will be prompted by the physiotherapist to check his standing position in the mirror. Still standing behind her patient with her hands on the brim of his pelvis, the physiotherapist asks him to rock slowly from side to side over his fixed base while she gives gentle pressure to control and guide his movement. She assists the movement laterally with a *forward* emphasis over the affected hip. It is practised as a swaying, rhythmical exercise and gradually the patient gains control and takes over the movement for himself.

Exercise 4: weight transfer over the affected hip with the affected leg placed forward. The exercise repeats Exercise 3 with the different starting position giving a new fixed base—affected leg placed forward one step, foot carefully positioned. The swaying movement (with assistance) again emphasises the lateral forward movement over the affected hip. At the same time, hip protraction must be maintained.

Exercise 5: control over a semi-flexed knee. The patient stands with both feet parallel and firmly on the floor but the sound foot is this time placed forward one step and both knees are slightly bent. The feet remain in their fixed position, heels in contact with the floor, and bilateral knee flexion and extension is practised—extension leading back into the starting position of mild flexion, that is, controlled movement over the semi-flexed knee. At this stage the affected knee will almost certainly need supporting assistance. The patient may also need supporting assistance for the affected arm. In this case the physiotherapist will sit behind her patient so that she can offer the necessary assistance using both of her hands and both of her knees. With one hand she supports the position of the affected hand on the bars, with the other she assists the necessary maintenance of pelvic protraction and she positions her legs to support his knee posteriorly and anteriorly. For example, if she is supporting his left knee, she places her left knee on the posterior aspect of his knee and uses her lower right leg to support his lower left leg anteriorly. He frequently does not need this maximum supporting assistance and she will have a hand free to give anterior knee support. She remains sitting, again using her knee for posterior support. She gradually withdraws her support and the patient takes over the movement for himself.

The patient is now able to weight-bear on both legs. This stage has been reached in the parallel bars by:

(a) Careful positioning of the *head* which is followed automatically by trunk alignment.

(b) Careful positioning of the *foot* which gives weight-bearing through the heel.

(c) Careful positioning of the *pelvis* to give weight-bearing through a controlled hip.

(d) Careful positioning of the *knee*, giving supporting assistance to prevent hyperextension.

(e) At no time forgetting the need for careful positioning of the affected arm and never allowing the shoulder to hang in internal rotation.

However, the knee may still be unstable and *must be* thoroughly stabilised to achieve the aim of restoring a normal walking pattern and the patient's return to a full and normal life. (Figure 60 shows a useful knee re-education position which is included in the exercise section using the plinth).

Exercise 6: alternate leg lifting on and off a low step. A wooden step is placed on the floor in front of the patient and the parallel bars are raised to a suitable height to allow him to reach forward and grasp them at shoulder level. Where the affected arm has not yet recovered sufficiently to maintain the position, it is suggested that the patient and the step face the bar on his sound side obliquely. He will then grasp the bar with both hands, the affected hand first with the sound hand placed firmly on top of it. In this way the required arm position with extended elbow and good shoulder protraction is easily maintained. The physiotherapist corrects the position of the affected leg and hip, not allowing hyperextension of the knee or retraction of the pelvis, while the patient lifts alternate legs on and off the step.

Exercise 7: control over a semi-flexed knee using the low step. The patient's exercise position is as for Exercise 6 except that the step is not placed obliquely. He grasps the bar on his sound side with his sound hand on top of his affected hand and places his sound leg on the step. In this position he reaches well forward on the rail of the parallel bars (as above), rotating his shoulders towards the sound side while he flexes the affected knee. The hands slide forward along the bar as the shoulders rotate. The physiotherapist gives any required supporting assistance to the knee and may assist pelvic protraction. To straighten up, the movement is reversed. The hands slide back as the shoulders rotate and the knee extends with supporting assistance. Decreasing amounts of supporting assistance will be given as control over the semi-flexed knee improves. *Note:* This exercise reduces hypertonicity in the leg, leads to controlled movement of the knee and makes a vital contribution to the restoration of normal leg function.

Exercise 8: stepping up and down. Alternate legs leading, stepping on and off a low step. The patient continues to hold the rail. Weight-bearing over the semi-flexed knee has been established. The patient lifts his sound leg forward onto the step and holds the position over two semi-flexed knees. The physiotherapist checks positioning. She then offers resistance to the forward knee, he straightens the leg and brings the affected leg up into position on the stool. He then flexes both knees and lifts the affected leg back on to the floor. The progression to leading with the affected leg will only follow when his affected knee is stabilised.

Exercise 9: stepping laterally on and off the low step is a useful exercise provided hip control is carefully maintained.

Exercise 10: knee flexion with hip extension of the affected leg while standing on the sound leg. The physiotherapist stands behind her patient while he watches his upright position with the help of the mirror. She uses one of her hands to control his hip while she gives assisted knee flexion with her other hand. Assisted knee flexion will lead to active knee flexion.

Exercise 11: Walking. Walking will only be practised in the parallel bars if it is carefully controlled with correct transfer of weight over the affected hip. Also, the affected hand must move forward along the bar— it *must not* be left behind to drag into internal rotation at the shoulder.

Note on walking rehabilitation: Where parallel bars are used for walking re-education, giving the patient support on his sound side, there is always the danger that he will cling to the sound side, lose the correct walking pattern which must include transfer of weight over the affected side, and his walking will quickly deteriorate into a compensatory walking pattern which depends on the sound side and thoroughly disrupts the rehabilitation programme. Personally, I do not use parallel bars for walking re-education; not unless they are used solely on the patient's affected side and he walks round the outside of the apparatus. At this stage it is thoroughly therapeutic to practise assisted walking with the patient if he clasps his hands (correctly positioned in front of his body) and the physiotherapist walks behind him giving supporting control to his pelvis. She assists pelvic protraction and lateral transfer of weight over the affected hip to give the correct walking pattern and she adds considerably to his self-confidence. This may be done in the bars— the bars will not be touched but will add the feeling of security that some patients need to regain the necessary self-confidence to go it alone. Where walking is concerned, the parallel bars should be left behind as soon as possible. Approached in this way, independent controlled walking is not hard to achieve.

Use of the plinth

Knee control. The importance of regaining knee control is by now fully understood. It is as important as regaining elbow control which has been emphasised all the way through the treatment programme. *Elbow control and knee control* must be rehabilitated together and neither allowed to lag behind. A treatment plinth with adjustable height is a very necessary piece of equipment but, where this is not available, steps of variable height must be used to raise the level of the patient's foot, or feet, to gain the required starting position for specific exercises.

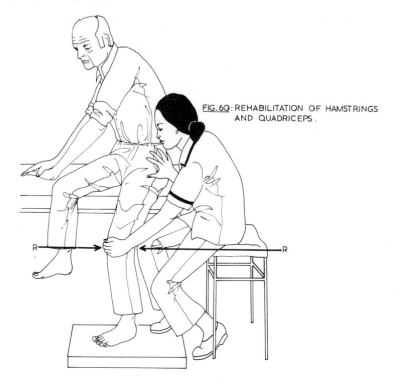

FIG.60: REHABILITATION OF HAMSTRINGS AND QUADRICEPS.

Figure 60, rehabilitation of hamstrings and quadriceps, illustrates a useful exercise position using the treatment plinth. As illustrated, a plinth with adjustable height was not available. A polystyrene block has been placed under the patient's affected foot to give the semi-flexed knee position necessary for the exercise. Note the position of the patient's arms. He leans on his hands to strengthen his knee against resistance offered by the physiotherapist's knee and again, because the arm is being used to weight-bear in the correct position, arm and leg rehabilitation is moving forward simultaneously. A progression is made when the patient learns to use the exercise as a means of 'walking' forward and backward along the edge of the plinth on the affected foot. Again he is weight-bearing over a semi-flexed knee. It is an equally good arm exercise. Where an adjustable plinth is not available, a longer polystyrene block would be necessary.

Figure 61 has been included as a reminder of the stages rehabilitation has been following. By now the patient ought to be able to do the following:

(a) Recognise the limb's position in space
(b) Support and hold the limb in space
(c) Move the limb in space.

If assessment shows that his ability is lacking, the physiotherapist will go back, isolate his difficulty, and step up earlier intensive training accordingly. Continuing with the programme, assisted and active movements are given with the patient sitting on the end of the plinth. He may lie back to practise knee movement with the hip extended. While the legs are hanging free he should also practise transference of weight over alternate hips without hand support. His hands will be clasped in front of him. This gives a further advance in training of equilibrium responses.

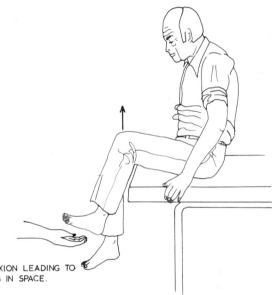

FIG.61: HIP AND KNEE FLEXION LEADING TO HOLDING THE LIMB IN SPACE.

Figure 62 shows stabilised forearm support on the plinth. As before, the thumbs and fingers should be abducted (particularly the thumbs). Where hand recovery is slow, particularly where hypertonicity is a problem, sponge rubber pieces may be used to hold the digits in abduction for all weight-bearing exercises. The inhibiting position with widely abducted fingers and thumb also helps to get round the difficulty of painful wrist extension. But I do not find this is necessary where correct rehabilitation procedures have been undertaken from the early days. (Note that the same technique may be applied to a neglected foot, widely abducted digits inhibiting spasm and allowing the forefoot to clear the ground in walking.) As shown in Figure 62, manual pressure is given to increase approximation from shoulder to elbow. Note the correct parallel position of the forearms. While in this position the patient will also practise rocking backwards and forwards over his forearms and he will transfer his weight from side to side. He is also in a

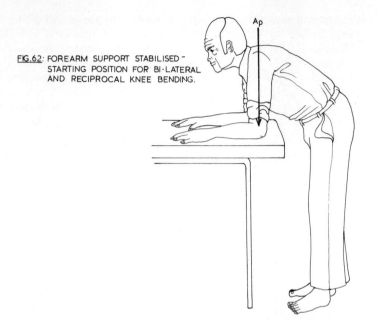

FIG.62: FOREARM SUPPORT STABILISED — STARTING POSITION FOR BI-LATERAL AND RECIPROCAL KNEE BENDING.

very good position for practising bilateral and reciprocal knee bending. Again all exercises are simultaneously rehabilitating arm and leg.

Figure 63 shows approximation of shoulder to hand with the position stabilised. If necessary supporting assistance is given to the elbow while tonic neck reflexes are stimulated. Resistance is used to increase extensor tone in the arms symmetrically and then asymmetrically to strengthen the weak arm. The arm position is very important. The patient is weight-bearing from the heel of his hand through an extended elbow to an externally rotated shoulder. His thumb is abducted and, if necessary, the physiotherapist will give hand support as in Figure 7f. Treatment is now moving into the area of hand recovery. The stroke patient must continue with the rocking movement over his hands that he began in crawling exercises. Unless he establishes this arm position as in Figure 63, and learns to rock backwards and forwards over an extended wrist, he will not free the primitive flexor grip and release his hands for functional movement. If this stage in arm rehabilitation gives trouble, the amount of time spent daily exercising while wearing an orally inflated pressure splint must be increased. The arm splint *must* be applied with the arm fully in the recovery pattern (including thumb and finger abduction) and inflated to the full amount the human lungs can achieve. The exercise session *must* include wrist extension with manual pressure to give approximation from the heel of the hand to the shoulder against counter pressure which is applied through a protracted shoulder. The exercise may be practised as in Figure 34 *but* firmer

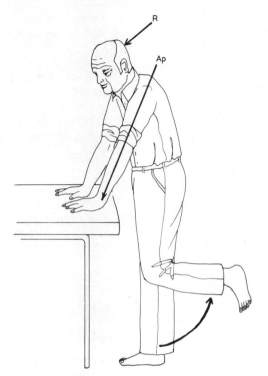

FIG.63: APPROXIMATION SHOULDER TO HAND: CONTROL OF THE LEG IN SPACE.

control is achieved if the wrist extension is applied as in Figure 36 and a second operator is available to give counter pressure through the protracted shoulder. Remember that the second operator may also make use of tonic neck reflexes. The exercise may also be practised in the supine position which makes it possible to *lean* hard on the palm of the hand but (a) the shoulder position must be well supported for counter pressure with the help of the second operator, and (b) the legs must be carefully positioned in the recovery pattern. The physiotherapist will use the exercise position she herself finds most suitable to give her the desired *strong* approximation through the correctly positioned limb. The patient with marked loss of muscle tone and hemianaesthesia will also continue his daily session of intermittent pressure with the pressure pump. Using this regime the most satisfactory results are achieved. As soon as the patient is weight-bearing from the heel of his hand through an extended elbow to an externally rotated shoulder—as in Figure 63— he is ready to continue with the rehabilitation programme. He will practise rocking forward over his hands in this position and this will lead him on to the final stages in arm rehabilitation. Again, he will also practise leg exercises while he leans on (and over) his hands. In a later progression he will stand at the end of the plinth in this position and lean over his hands using strong lumbrical action so that he leans on his finger-tips through extended and abducted fingers. I find this exercise re-establishes the spherical grip and opposition of thumb to little finger.

The plinth has other uses—for example, it is suitable for lateral haunch walking with the lower legs hanging free and for exercises in stand kneeling and side sitting—but the physiotherapist will plan her own treatment programme. The purpose here is to state the principles of rehabilitation and to give a fairly simple outline of possible exercises. Obviously all the possible exercises cannot be given.

Revision of techniques that lead to controlled walking

All the way through the rehabilitation programme the importance of correct positioning has been stressed. Whatever the state of muscle tone that is found to be present on careful assessment, the need for maintaining and using anti-spasm positioning and working within the anti-spasm pattern has at no time been forgotten. This is the only way to obtain the high standard of treatment with the consequent successful recovery rate that must be the physiotherapist's aim.

Next, sensory loss, hypotonicity and the tremendous hurdle placed in the way of recovery by the loss of—in particular—proprioceptive sense was considered and the 'anti-spasm' approach was continued. It became apparent why the word *recovery* might be more correctly used to describe positions and patterns of movement used in the treatment plan. The *anti-spasm* pattern and the *recovery* pattern were synonymous and in all stages of rehabilitation, while motor and sensory development progressed, movement kept well within this *recovery* pattern. While treatment continued to follow the same pattern as before, the urgent need to step up sensory input was discussed. Techniques for increasing sensory input were suggested, in particular deep pressure techniques were shown as a way of giving a dynamic boost to sensory loss. Techniques for increasing and decreasing muscle tone were also suggested—the appropriate measures to be taken according to assessment findings.

In the broad treatment plan under discussion, the patient is now ready to begin controlled walking.

In all cases, weight-bearing through the affected limbs is vital to recovery; this means, gravity approximation, gravity approximation increased by manual pressure and full weight-bearing—all taking place through a *correctly positioned base.* This base will either be the hand or the foot. Where correct positioning is not used (and correct positioning must include weight-bearing over a correctly positioned base) there is a failure to recognise perhaps the most important fundamental principle on which rehabilitation is based.

Standing on the hand—or weight-bearing from hand to shoulder—is always carried out with the thumb and fingers widely abducted and weight is transmitted through an externally rotated shoulder and an extended elbow and wrist to the heel of the hand.

Standing on the foot must never allow a badly positioned foot. Weight must be taken through the heel with the whole foot carefully positioned on the floor, parallel to the sound foot and not externally rotated. Assistance must be given with foot positioning for standing in the early days. Weight-bearing over the semi-flexed knee, as shown is an important part of leg rehabilitation. As already stated, assisted abduction of the toes (using small sponge rubber pads to separate the toes) should be added where adequate treatment was not started in the early days and spasm has been allowed to develop.

The whole rehabilitation programme is based on redevelopment of controlled movement in response to reflex activity. When weight is distributed through correctly positioned limbs to the heel of the hand and the heel of the foot, reflex response is at its optimum and postural mechanisms are reinforced to make weight-bearing possible. This is why *the base must be correct.*

If *equilibrium responses* have not been fully redeveloped on the affected side the patient will have difficulty in:

(a) placing his limbs
(b) holding his limbs at rest and against gravity, and
(c) maintaining his balance.

Equilibrium responses include the necessary shifts in muscle tone with compensating movements to allow us to accomodate for any altering situation caused by changes of position or environment. When fully developed, equilibrium responses allow us to support our weight over a fixed base, to prop over a fixed base while reaching out in any direction, to maintain balance against an external opposing force or to regain balance by reaching out, by hopping, or by side-stepping. It must be remembered, *these responses develop from righting reflexes* and are *basal* responses which are part *cortical*—they are variable and can be overruled at cortical level—*but* must be established before cortical level can be effective.

Thus, if the patient is found to have difficulty in supporting his weight over his fixed base in any stage of the treatment programme (which is leading him towards supporting his weight in standing) he must be taken back to his earlier training and the previous stage (or missing link), must be thoroughly established remembering that all stages overlap and none must be omitted.

Righting reflexes and equilibrium responses, when they are properly understood by the physiotherapist, must lead her to use the correct and effective techniques that will re-establish deficit fairly quickly. She uses rolling, rolling to sitting, rolling to propping, crawling and kneeling and thoroughly stabilises all positions. Each progression makes a greater demand and so leads forward.

For example, study Figure 50, full kneeling, transferring weight over the affected side. This exercise shows that the patient is able to support his weight over his affected hand and knee while he moves his sound hand and knee. At this stage some physiotherapists may choose to train 'magnet' responses. To give an example, this simply means that the patient (as in Fig. 50) will keep both knees on the floor and lift his sound hand to place his finger-tips against his physiotherapist's finger-tips. He is taught to maintain finger-tip contact and follow her hand movements. He is supporting his weight over a fixed base while reaching out in any direction. Where equilibrium responses have failed to be fully established this technique has a place in the rehabilitation programme but it must be used intelligently, the physiotherapist not allowing her enthusiasm to run away with her. It can fail badly if the patient is allowed to overbalance frequently and shatter his self-confidence. All exercise must encourage and not defeat the patient and this rule is particularly true when treatment is offered to stroke patients. The use of a wall mirror (full-length) can be helpful here. Still kneeling, correctly positioned as in Figure 50, the patient balances on both knees and the affected hand (elbow support given if necessary) and extends his neck to look in the mirror, lifts his sound hand, reaches to gain mirror finger-tip contact and moves his hand from side to side, maintaining finger-tip contact with the mirror and balancing over his affected arm. The exercise stays in one plane but assists in establishing lateral balance, or equilibrium response. Note that the thicker and softer the floor mattress the greater the demand—and therefore the greater the response. Understandably, then, training in 'magnet responses' will not be undertaken very early in the treatment plan.

I would make the same comment about the use of Freeman's balance board. The use of an unstable base has an important part to play, but the unstable base must be introduced in the right place, not too early in the treatment programme. Normal responses will be obtained if the patient is introduced to an unstable base in exactly the same way as an infant might be given this altering situation (if he is to cope with it successfully). He must feel secure. A baby that has just learnt to sit up would not be expected to sit on anything quite so insecure as a Freeman's balance board. He might be expected to maintain his balance if he was placed on a sponge rubber cushion or mattress. So again, modelling the treatment plan on the development of the infant, there is a place for (indeed, there is a need for) use of the unstable base but it must be used intelligently. To sum up, the floor mattress should be large, soft and springy. The suitable chair ought to have a flat, square, springy rubber cushion, the table for forearm support ought to have a thick, springy surface which provides a mildly unstable base and the necessary friction to prevent the limb from sliding. The rocking chair ought to be used and the Freeman's balance board ought not to be introduced until the later stages of equilibrium training.

Figure 64 shows a piece of apparatus that may also be introduced to

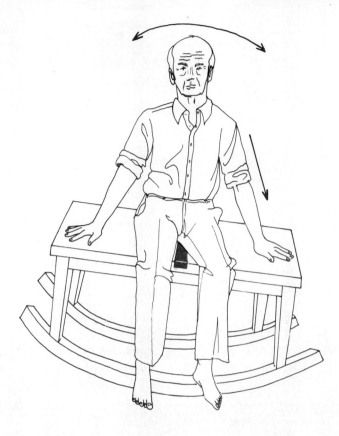

FIG.64: LATERAL ROCKING.

advantage, but again not too early in the treatment programme. It should be used to facilitate equilibrium responses when sitting balance has been thoroughly stabilised and, if necessary, elbow support will be given. In other words, it will be used when the patient feels safe enough on this type of unstable base to enjoy his treatment. As illustrated the patient's feet hang free and not enough care has been taken with hip positioning. I also find a similar stool on lower rockers (where the patient's feet are positioned on the floor) of tremendous value. In this case, a lateral lean to the affected side so that weight is distributed over a meticulously positioned hand and foot makes a demand that gains a thoroughly therapeutic response.

Restoration of equilibrium responses leads to controlled walking.

Controlled walking
  Figure 65, controlled walking, as illustrated, shows walking which is

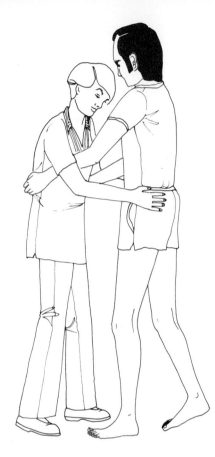

FIG.65: CONTROLLED WALKING.

controlled by the physiotherapist from the patient's pelvic level. The method illustrated is useful for a nervous patient who is in the early stages of walking re-education. It gives him something to hold onto while his affected arm is maintained in a good position. The physiotherapist may grip his forearms with her upper arms while, at the same time, she gives supporting pelvic control. This walking exercise may also be practised with the patient's arms placed up on the physiotherapist's shoulders, or she may walk behind her patient giving supporting pelvic control from behind while he walks with his hands clasped at the front. Again, in all three of these possible supporting positions, the pelvic controlled assistance emphasises the lateral forward movement over the affected hip.

Figure 66 gives a very useful supporting hold for the initial sessions in training of controlled walking. This diagram illustrates my own particu-

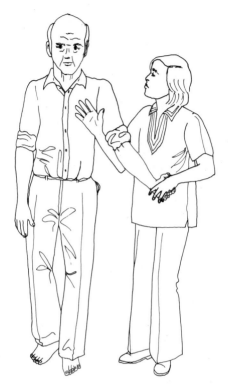

FIG. 66: A USEFUL HOLD TO CONTROL WALKING.

lar favourite supporting hold for walking the stroke patient. The patient's affected arm is well positioned, weight being transferred from the externally rotated shoulder down through an extended elbow to the heel of the hand. Note the handshake grip (Fig. 7a or b) the physiotherapist gives to her patient, keeping his thumb uppermost to maintain external rotation of the shoulder. With her other hand she extends her wrist, thumb and fingers (with abduction) to give maximum hand contact with his lateral chest wall and the anterior aspect of his shoulder while she maintains his elbow extension with her upper arm. This puts her in an ideal position to control his body movement and assist in correct transfer of weight as he walks. I find that where this position is used, and no other, controlled walking is quickly established and correct weight transfer does not usually give any trouble. Here the very tall physiotherapist is at a disadvantage. *Walking should never be led from the patient's sound side.*

Where the full rehabilitation programme has been faithfully carried out, this latter supporting position for assisted walking (Fig. 66) very quickly leads into controlled walking where the patient has established a normal gait, secure balance and complete independence. If I were to criticise the artist's diagram I might suggest that the physiotherapist ought to be a little closer to her patient if she is to have absolute control over any movement he makes. Her right hand is placed forward, up, and under his arm, giving a pivot which she uses as her central point of control. This is why it is not so easy for a tall operator to control the movement as effectively as a small person, particularly if the patient is short.

To say that *walking should never be led from the sound side* is simply to make a statement that follows the way of thinking that is set out in this book. That is, that the correct and only approach when handling the stroke patient is the approach that is made from his affected side.

The correct approach, then, will be understood to mean that the patient will be approached from his affected side and he will use his sound arm and the sound half of his body almost entirely in exercises which involve *cross facilitation—working with the sound side* **across** *the midline to the affected side to initiate bilateral activity.* Walking leads to turning round and the question that is often asked: 'Which way does the patient turn?' This ought not to cause any confusion if the correct approach is understood. Following the obvious rehabilitation sequence, he will turn into—or towards—the affected side, cross facilitating over the midline. The affected side becomes the pivot and he turns round it, transferring weight through the affected leg and making one more forward step in his rehabilitation. Turning should be undertaken slowly and deliberately until it becomes an established and reliable manoeuvre.

The wrong approach will be understood to mean that the patient will be approached from his sound side. His visitors will sit on his sound side, his locker or table will be placed on his sound side, the television set will be positioned on his sound side and those who care for him will approach him from his sound side. He will be expected to help himself by using his sound side and *working with the sound side* **away from** *midline and the affected side. To do this is to offer rehabilitation that will effectively put an end to successful rehabilitation of the affected side.* This approach inevitably leads to the unsatisfactory result; that is, to the patient who has compensated for his disability with his sound side and who remains half of his former self, or less than half of his former self because of resulting deformities. From the very first day of rehabilitation treatment, all those who handle the stroke patient ought to be aware of the danger of using the wrong approach.

The trouble is that in the early days it often seems quicker and easier—even more satisfactory at times—to allow, or to teach, the patient to compensate for his lost ability with his sound side. This easy way towards some sort of quick independence is a snare and a delusion, or a trap that must be avoided. Inadequate early independence gained by teaching a patient to compensate with his sound side can only reinforce abnormal patterns of movement and hasten the end picture of a permanently inadequate and deformed patient with wretched residual disability. The patient who is allowed to compensate with his sound side may walk again, but—if he succeeds in walking—he will do so with a leg held stiffly in extension while his arm remains a useless appendage and *he will never again initiate movement from his affected side.* He will become, at best, a member of the community who is trying to face normal living with the residual problem of this spastic gait plus a useless arm. Or, worse still, he may be forced to become an inmate of an institution because the door that ought to have led to more normal living was slammed in his face. He has joined the ranks of the severely disabled.

This simple difference in the two methods of approach to stroke rehabilitation cannot be stressed too often. There are still many who make the one-sided compensating approach to treatment which does the patient a great disservice. It is not helpful here to suggest that some patients recover whatever is done—or not done—for them. We are discussing the management of major strokes. If I repeat what I have said before, it is because it is most urgently necessary to get this message across. We, as physiotherapists, must lead the rehabilitation field.

Treatment aids

Walking aids ought not to be necessary if it has been possible to follow the symmetrical rehabilitation programme from the beginning. The treatment stages which have re-established postural reactions, re-educated lateral transfer of body weight over a correctly positioned foot and a semi-flexed knee, have led to controlled symmetrical walking. But if the patient has failed to reach the target of controlled balance over a correctly positioned foot with a stabilised knee and good pelvic position, treatment aids may be brought into use. It is now necessary to think in terms of proximal to distal weight transfer *with distal to proximal movement.* The test of full recovery of controlled selective movement is the final rehabilitation of the distal to proximal sequence.

Figure 67, the Arjo pilot, shows one of the most sophisticated walking aids on the market and it is proving its worth in many large physiotherapy departments which care for the severely disabled. Its special features include adjustable forearm rests which may be pumped up to the required height, or lowered by finger-tip pressure on a lever, locking wheels and solid dependability. In those departments which have an Arjo pilot as part of the equipment, it can be used for stroke rehabilitation most usefully. Here, the forearm rests and handgrips (as illustrated in Figure 67), make it possible to weight-bear on correctly positioned forearms in standing. The handgrips are vertical and the arm-rests parallel, giving the patient the forearm positioning which treatment has aimed to maintain for forearm weight-bearing since the first day he sat out of bed. Thus, if he stands in the Arjo pilot, he is in an ideal position to work at both arm and leg rehabilitation.

Figure 68, the gutter extension arm-rest ought perhaps to be mentioned here. It is a most useful gadget. It is made of plastic guttering, is

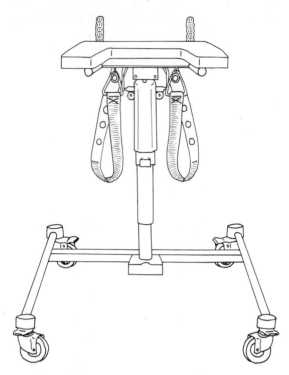

FIG.67: THE ARJO PILOT, A USEFUL REHABILITATION AID.

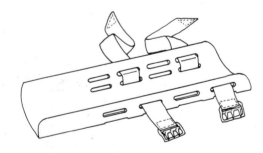

FIG.68: GUTTER EXTENSION ARM REST.

easily strapped to the appropriate arm-rest of the patient's chair and is adjustable in length by altering the position of the straps. If it is fastened to his chair, the patient ought to be taught to use it correctly for remedial exercise and to support his arm at any time his table is not immediately available. He rests his forearm *forward* on the support and is then well placed to practise elbow propping over a protracted and externally rotated shoulder and forearm leaning for cross facilitation, for example, reaching across midline with his sound hand towards his locker. As long as the need for shoulder to elbow approximation, cross facilitation, and forearm leaning with the necessity to maintain careful positioning continues (that is, as long as arm rehabilitation continues), the gutter extension arm-rest is a necessary treatment aid.

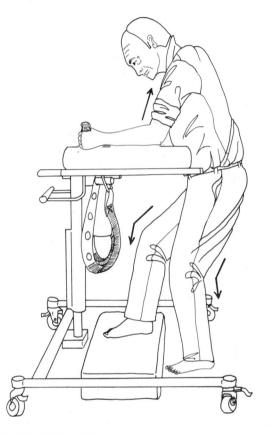

FIG.69: ARJO PILOT IN USE.

1) Forearm support.
2) Stepping up.
3) Control over semi - flexed knee.

Figure 69 shows the Arjo pilot in use. The groin straps will not be used for the stroke patient. The artist has produced an illustration which shows the forearm rests in use while the patient practises control over the semi-flexed knee with his sound leg placed on a low step. For steps, again I use a series of polystyrene blocks. They are light to lift and easily stored. In the position illustrated, the patient is ideally placed to practise left-sided lateral transfer of his body weight over forearm and hip. The left foot is correctly positioned and the physiotherapist can stand back and watch carefully to see if hip protraction is maintained. If the hip retracts on weight-bearing she will check the foot position again, making sure the heel is correctly placed. If he still fails to maintain a satisfactory position there are four points she should remember.

1. She will *position his head,* making use of tonic neck reflexes to reinforce underlying postural mechanisms.

2. She will again *check the foot position.*

3. She will *position his pelvis* and be ready to assist correct pelvic movement with manual pressure.

4. She will *stabilise the knee position* with one of her knees and one hand (as in Fig. 60).

She is then in a position to help him to practise the movement until he is able to maintain a satisfactory position unaided.

In the same position, using the polystyrene block and the Arjo pilot with the forearm rests a little higher, the patient may practise lateral weight transfer over the affected hip. In this position with the sound leg placed forward on the step, lateral transfer over the affected side demands *marked pelvic rotation.* While the patient transfers his weight over the semi-flexed knee, the physiotherapist will assist forward rotation of the pelvis on the affected side. She may also stabilise the knee as above and it goes without saying that the correct foot position is of first importance. If no Arjo pilot is available this exercise may be practised in the parallel bars.

Continuing to use the Arjo pilot with the patient positioned as in Figure 69, he is taught to step up on to the step, bringing the affected foot up beside the sound foot. To achieve this, the physiotherapist offers manual pressure to the forward knee and the patient stretches up over the sound foot and lifts the affected foot on to the step. He is taught to lean on his forearms and flex both knees before he steps down again. Note that the same exercise may be practised at the end of the plinth (as in Fig. 62) but this suggestion serves to illustrate the need for a plinth which is adjustable in height. As a later progression he will step up leading with the affected foot.

Forearm support in the Arjo pilot will also be used to practise bilateral and reciprocal knee bending. The above suggestions show what a useful piece of apparatus this is for stroke rehabilitation. It may finally be used to establish controlled walking. It also has a detachable seat which is not included in the diagram because it was not used in this particular series of exercises. As shown in Figure 69, the groin straps are slung up out of the way and the wheel brakes are all four on.

Note: The use of a quadruped or tripod walking aid in the sound hand will only serve to encourage compensation with the sound side, will actively prevent normal weight transfer over the affected side and will reinforce the resulting abnormal stance.

Final stages in arm rehabilitation

The final stages in arm rehabilitation can only be undertaken when controlled shoulder and elbow movement have been re-established—the patient will be able to place his limb and hold it in space because adequate normal tone has been re-established and muscles have been strengthened by active exercise.

Summary of the treatment plan that has been followed and which has led to controlled shoulder and elbow movement whatever the state of muscle tone that was found to be present on careful assessment.

Muscle tone. Because there are always changes in normal muscle tone in stroke patients, the state of tone was assessed with great care.

Increased muscle tone. Where increased muscle tone (hypertonicity or spasticity) was found to be present, the arm drifted into the synergic pattern of tonic contraction and was resistant to passive movement into the anti-spasm, or *recovery* pattern *plus elevation.* The patient had lost his ability to maintain his limb in space in any position because of excessive tone in the anti-gravity muscles.

Decreased muscle tone. Where decreased muscle tone (hypotonicity or flaccidity) was found to be present, the arm was limp and flabby and could not be supported in space, that is in the anti-gravity position, because of muscle weakness. It felt heavy when moved passively into the *recovery* pattern plus elevation. Treatment, therefore, had to include techniques to decrease or to increase muscle tone as necessary.

Increased muscle tone. Where increased muscle tone was found, treatment included:

1. Positioning.
2. Pressure splints (orally inflated) to inhibit dominant reflexes.
3. Passive movements.
4. Assisted movements.
5. Active assisted movements.
6. Tapping (or prodding) on appropriate surfaces to prevent drifting.
7. Active assisted movements and holding in space (with pressure splint inhibiting dominant reflexes).
8. Active movements and holding in space (with pressure splint inhibiting dominant reflexes).
9. Active movements and holding in space.
10. Active resisted movements. (Resistance is *never* given in early treatment but must be used in arm re-education as soon as a fair degree of shoulder control has been established. In this case dominant reflexes are firmly inhibited by a pressure splint which is applied in the full inhibiting pattern and the legs are positioned at the same time with meticulous care.)
11. Weight-bearing over a correctly positioned base.

Decreased muscle tone. Where decreased muscle tone was found, treatment included:

1. Positioning.

2. Pressure splint (orally inflatable) to support flaccid limb for shoulder exercise.

3. Pressure splint (orally inflatable) to give sustained deep and superficial pressure on correctly positioned limb while movement within the tissues is stimulated (e.g. rolling from side to side, position as in Fig. 35).

4. Approximation of joint surfaces (with supporting assistance of orally inflatable pressure splint) to facilitate underlying postural mechanisms.

5. Active assisted movements (with supporting pressure splint).

6. Active assisted movement and holding in space (with supporting pressure).

7. Tapping (or pounding) of the heel of the hand (or foot) with the limb in the recovery pattern.

8. Active movement and holding in space.

9. Active resisted movements. (Resistance is never given in early treatment as above.)

10. Weight-bearing over a correctly positioned base.

Intermittent pressure, using a pressure pump, was given for one hour daily to further step up sensory input where proprioceptive loss was present. The aim was to bombard the proprioceptors to activate the anterior horn cells.

No two patients are exactly the same and the physiotherapist *must* assess the patient's tonal state correctly and alter and adjust the treatment plan according to her findings. The skill of the physiotherapist lies in her ability to assess and understand the problems each patient presents so that she may offer the specialised care he so urgently needs. The greatest need for the spastic limb is to *inhibit the drift into the spastic pattern* and to teach limb control via passive to active exercise. The greatest need for the flaccid limb is to *support with deep pressure* to allow approximation and weight-bearing through a correctly placed limb, to increase muscle tone, to stimulate proprioceptors and to reinforce underlying postural mechanisms. The skill lies in combining these two needs to fit the co-existing symptoms. Thus, while fitting the treatment programme to the symptoms, and altering the techniques to meet the need, all treatment follows the same broad pattern.

The final stages of rehabilitating *controlled movement of the hand can only be obtained by freeing the hand from the primitive flexor grasp and developing controlled movement from distal to proximal.*

Going back again in the rehabilitation programme, it is wise to pick out the *essential* measures that have been taken to achieve the full arm rehabilitation that will leave no residual disability for the unfortunate patient to bear. For many years, with a careful and correct approach to stroke rehabilitation, it has been possible to achieve perfect leg function. The following points, singled out of the broad treatment plan, ought to lead to equally satisfactory results in the affected arm.

1. As always, careful positioning in the recovery pattern must be maintained at all times.

2. The patient must not be asked to lead an activity with an area of disability until muscle tone has been restored.

3. Until muscle tone has been restored, forearm support should be given at all times by using a table or extended gutter support.

4. The patient should, therefore, not be allowed to use his hand *in any way* without forearm support until he can place his arm in space and hold it there.

5. Constant repetition of approximation with manual pressure from the heel of the hand through an extended elbow to an externally rotated shoulder must be given. It will be practised with an orally inflated pressure splint on the arm. An assistant is asked to support the shoulder firmly in protraction and to give the necessary counter pressure. In the later stages of rehabilitation it may be practised without the aid of the splint.

6. The patient must be taught to balance in the crawling position on hands and knees with extended elbows. He must rock backwards and forwards over his hands to begin *the* vital exercise to free the primitive flexor grasp and develop controlled hand movements.

7. The patient should be taught to use every opportunity to balance over extended elbows with correctly positioned hands placed on the arms of a chair, on a plinth, on a table or on any suitable surface. *He must stand on his hands.*

Failure to establish any one of these progressions will lead to failure to establish precision movements of the hand. The progressions move from forearm propping support, to hand propping support with the aid of a splint, to restored muscle tone, to hand propping support without the aid of a splint, to standing on the correctly positioned hand and rocking over the fixed base. It can be seen that where arm rehabilitation follows this plan it is very similar to the rehabilitation plan that has been followed for the leg. This is the aim. It has long been thought that leg rehabilitation depends on weight-bearing over a correctly positioned foot. After the necessary preliminary treatment that leads up to standing, if the base is correctly placed the patient will stand. In the same way, arm rehabilitation depends on standing on the hand, or weight-bearing over a correctly positioned hand. Again, after the preliminary treatment that leads up to standing on the hand, if the base is correctly placed the patient will support his weight over his hand. The hand must maintain a comfortable degree of external rotation and thumb and fingers must be abducted with the wrist extended. Weight will be distributed through the heel of the hand.

Later stages of leg rehabilitation showed the importance of establishing strong knee control and correct foot positioning for standing. Later stages of arm rehabilitation will have the same priorities. Elbow control must be thoroughly established.

FINAL STAGES IN ARM REHABILITATION.

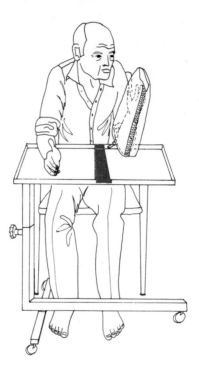

FIG.70: ELBOW FLEXION.

Figure 70 shows the patient sitting at a table with elbows supported in a good working position for arm rehabilitation. (His feet are properly placed flat on the floor. If the patient does not by now automatically position his leg he must be corrected if he sits badly). As shown in Figure 70, the patient is practising reciprocal elbow flexion and extension. He is taught to move both arms together and when he has mastered the exercise he is taught to use alternate arms. Next he is taught a sequence of movement—both hands followed immediately by alternate hands, sound hand leading. Inability to flex the elbow must not be allowed to persist. Where there is any difficulty, patients frequently find the support of a pressure splint *for hand and wrist* (as illustrated) holding the thumb and fingers in the inhibiting position is all that is needed to control dominant reflexes and make movement possible. This leads to the ability to perform the movement against resistance with the splint on. The physiotherapist will give approximation from shoulder to elbow by manual pressure while the patient sits in this position. She will also use bone tapping over the extensor surface of the elbow joint by grasping the pressure splint and lifting it up and down to tap the elbow firmly down on the table. This will be followed by elbow extension against resistance. All exercises must then be established with the splint off.

Note: The patient should now be beginning to think in terms of hand movement and of leading arm movement with his hand—the distal to proximal sequence. Prior to this it is frequently found that movement will be facilitated by asking the patient to think of any specific movement as taking place in the joint concerned. For example: 'Think about your elbow . . . Look at your elbow . . . Help me to bend your elbow . . .' will gain a response that may fail if the command given is: 'Take your hand up to your mouth.' Or, in some cases, a response will be gained by the command: 'Look at your hand . . . Take your mouth down to meet your hand. . .' The patient 'thinks' the movement, moves his head and asymmetrical neck flexion brings in the tonic neck reflex. The physiotherapist must at all times use her skill to devise ways and means of gaining the response she requires and she must make use of every sensory cue that is available, using voice, touch and vision to maximum effect. She will always fit her commands to suit each new situation so that she gains a response. The same old routine work out, day after day, with the same mechanical commands given in a dull voice must have no part in stroke rehabilitation.

Figure 62 will serve to illustrate the next important exercise which must be thoroughly established—*controlled weight-bearing over the hands while flexing and extending the elbows.* Consult Figure 62 and then change the starting position slightly so that the patient's elbows are drawn back to the edge of the plinth and his fingers are more widely abducted. From this position he does hand press-ups—he pushes down on his hands and extends his elbows to weight-bear over his hands before he returns to the starting position. The hands remain firmly in place. This means that he is practising weight-bearing through a controlled elbow to a correctly positioned base. He is doing with his arm what he has already done with his leg. He learns to weight-bear over a semi-flexed elbow. Where necessary, supporting assistance will be given to the elbow and sponge rubber pieces may be used to assist finger abduction, but all support must be withdrawn as soon as possible. Active exercise over controlled elbows will lead to resisted exercise over controlled elbows. This exercise will serve to illustrate just how dynamic the treatment must be if the arm is to be re-educated to its former ability and the patient is to regain a skilled and useful hand.

Figure 71 shows wrist extension with the hand and wrist pressure splint on. This exercise is used where wrist extension is limited and/or painful. Wrist extension will be practised at first as a manipulation, the relaxation given by a correctly applied splint making the manipulation pain free. Maintaining the position, approximation by manual pressure from the heel of the hand to the elbow may be given. An assistant will be

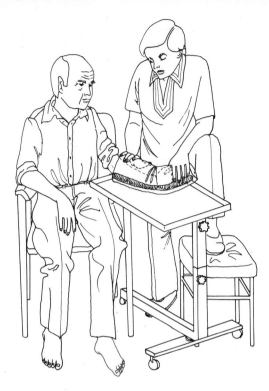

FIG.71: WRIST EXTENSION.

asked to give counter-pressure behind the elbow. Both of these manipu-
lations ought to be practised until the patient can weight-bear on a fully
extended pain free wrist. If, at this stage, the wrist gives trouble, turn
back to Figures 34 and 36 and decide, for future reference, if this section
of treatment was adequately covered.

Figure 72, rotation, is included as a reminder that loss of rotation will
be found where hypertonicity is a problem. If the programme of
treatment as given here has been followed, it should not be a problem,
but it will still be necessary to practise rotation as a controlled voluntary
action and, at this stage, with forearm support. Weak muscles must be
strengthened. Also, where hypotonicity is found, techniques to increase
muscle tone must still be used and, where necessary, sensory input must
be stepped up in every possible way. It is necessary to practise every
exercise with great care. The patient will be encouraged to use his eyes to
step up sensory input. He will use both forearms, as in Figure 72, and he
will be taught to use the affected hand to mimic the movement made by
the sound hand. Inability to rotate can be the hurdle that prevents a
satisfactory return to controlled hand movement.

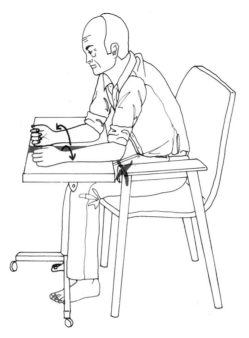

FIG. 72 : ROTATION .

If the patient is faced with the problem of inability to rotate satısfac-
torily it will be helpful to ask him to maintain positioning (as in Fig. 72)
and then clasp his hands, fingers interlaced and palms touching. He now
uses the sound hand to lead the affected hand into pronation and
supination. He establishes the movement as an active assisted movement for the affected hand and he is taught to progress (still with hands
clasped) to active movement and then to resisted movement.

Maintaining the same position (as in Fig. 72 but still with hands
clasped) he will practise wrist flexion and extension in the same way—
assisted movement leading to resisted movement.

Finally he will unlace his fingers and, keeping palms and fingers
pressed firmly together, fingers and thumbs abducted, he will again
practise wrist flexion and extension until it becomes a controlled
exercise he can perform against resistance offered by his sound hand.
Still with hands pressed firmly together in this attitude of prayer (but
with thumbs and fingers abducted) he will separate his palms so that his
finger-tips remain in contact and he will press thumbs and finger-tips
firmly together. He is now getting down to the final work on finger
control.

Elbow flexion and extension, forearm pronation and supination,
wrist flexion and extension and finger flexion and extension will all be
practised frequently as free exercise. Finger flexion and extension will

next be used as grasp and release in an exercise to pick up objects. Where rehabilitation has *not* been carried out sufficiently to free the primitive flexor grip and release the hand for functional movement, the patient will be able to grasp an article but he will not be able to release it. In this case, the exercise programme must go right back to weight-bearing over the hand in the crawling position and continue from there. For the final stages in grasp/release training, I use two very light balls made of plastic foam and about four inches in diameter (ten centimetres) for the average sized male hand. The patient is taught to pick up the ball very carefully with a spherical finger-tip grip, move it slowly through space, hold it in space and place it on an indicated spot. This exercise demands a fair degree of control, including a mass finger movement that is bordering on precision control. When it is achieved satisfactorily the end of arm rehabilitation and a return to normal living is in view. I use two balls in bilateral exercise before attempting to use one as above. All of these bilateral hand exercises in the final stages of arm rehabilitation have been done with elbow support, or forearm support, or both. The final exercise listed using one ball in the affected hand has been done without support.

The patient is now ready to continue developing controlled hand movements and to lead into activities which use the hand freely and without support of any kind. This is because the patient can now place his arm in space and hold it there and he has fully developed controlled movement from shoulder to elbow to hand. He has also freed the primitive flexor grip and released his hand for functional movement. He has *restored muscle tone* and is developing controlled hand movements which will now include the use of his hands to lead activities in the final sequence of distal to proximal control. He should no longer require supporting assistance or supervision in positioning and placing to gain the desired response. This does not mean that he will stop all previous exercise. He must continue to weight-bear over controlled knees and controlled elbows with correctly positioned feet and hands, he must continue a reasonable daily scheme of exercise and he must go ahead with the final stages in rehabilitation. Weak muscles must be strengthened and lost skill regained. The most demanding task is still ahead of him. He is going to return to normal living.

For continued arm rehabilitation, if he has not already done so, the patient ought to transfer to a large table, preferably a table with a polished surface and the height must be right. Figure 72 illustrates the need for a larger table. The diagram shows bad positioning in that the elbow is not supported—otherwise the height of the table is correct and the patient's position is good.

Sitting at a large table, the patient may be left to practise a sequence of simple exercises by himself—*but* he must not be allowed to build up *frustration* because he is given repetitive little tasks which irritate him in a sequence he cannot remember. He will sit, using both hands with elbows and ulna borders of his forearms resting on the table and forearms parallel. This will be his starting position and he will return to it between exercises. If he is tolerant of the idea he will be given a simple routine at first. This will include:

1. Making fists.
2. Rotating.
3. Elbow flexion and extension.
4. Wrist flexion and extension.
5. Hands pressed together in an attitude of prayer with thumbs and fingers abducted, wrist flexion and extension, sound hand assisting movement.
6. As 5 with sound hand resisting movement.
7. As 5 with palms separated and finger-tips pressed together.
8. Leaning over forearms, hands fixed palms down and digits abducted pulling and pushing.
9. Sliding: palms placed over suitable size of Sellotape tin, finger-tip grip, sliding tins in all directions.
10. Precision movements including small grip as in tower building with small blocks of wood, or pinch grip as in handling coloured pencil.
11. Selecting plastic cups of diminishing size from random lay out and placing one inside the other.
12. Selecting plastic cups of increasing size from random lay out and building tower.
13. Using *Theraplast:* a modelling material which will encourage the use of both hands as well as facilitating full rehabilitation of the affected hand.

Note: Exercises given must be chosen with care. For example, numbers 11 and 12 would not be given as a hand exercise where assessment has shown diminished learning ability, disturbance of interpretation of spatial relationships, apraxia or agnosia to be present (consult the chapter on assessment).

Theraplast (or modelling material), *and the final stages of hand rehabilitation.*

Theraplast should be readily obtainable from the medical suppliers for occupational therapy needs. Plasticine may also be used but I have a personal preference for Theraplast. It does not smell unpleasantly, it is clean to use and makes a more satisfactory functional demand. A suitable modelling material ought to be included as a necessary aid in rehabilitation of precision movements of the hand. It must not remain the prerogative of the occupational therapist to use this aid. This point illustrates very nicely how important it is for the therapists (physio and occupational) to maintain no more than a very flexible dividing line between departments and to cooperate fully over treatment. It is, for instance, vitally important for *both* therapists to understand that, in the stroke patient, no activity will be led—or will be expected to be led—by an area of disability until muscle tone has been restored. For example, in the early days, the patient should not be expected to *hold* a cup of tea using *both* hands with the affected arm in slings. The hand and arm pattern would at once turn in to the pattern dictated by uninhibited dominant reflexes. At this stage it is important to remember that static reflexes are not integrated into controlled movement. Thus, making excessive demands and encouraging early, willed, voluntary effort all serve to stimulate unwanted dominant reflex activity and must be discarded from any treatment programme.

With restored muscle tone and controlled shoulder and elbow movement, the patient is ready to rehabilitate the hand with the help of both the physio and the O.T. It is quite wrong to call on the O.T's. help too early in the programme or to exclude the physio from this final vital step in full rehabilitation.

The uses of Theraplast for hand rehabilitation:

1. *In the early stages of rehabilitation.* Where any patient has difficulty in maintaining the handclasp position, fingers interlaced, palms touching, Theraplast can be used to advantage. The patient is given a piece of thoroughly softened and moulded Theraplast to squash between his palms and the heels of his hands. It acts as a visual and sensory reminder to keep his palms and the heels of his hands firmly in contact. Plasticine is more useful at this stage.

2. *In the intermediary stages of rehabilitation.* Theraplast may be used to facilitate weight-bearing through a correctly positioned hand. With the shoulder externally rotated, elbow and wrist extended, the affected hand is placed firmly on a flattened piece of Theraplast (fingers and thumb abducted). After leaning over this correctly positioned base, the imprint must show firm weight-bearing through the heel of the hand.

3. *In the final stages of rehabilitation.* Precision movements of the hand must be established in the final stages of rehabilitation. The patient has followed through all the necessary steps which lead to freeing of his flexor grip and releasing of his hand for functional movement. In other words, primitive reflex movement has been restored to controlled movement, but this movement is frequently poor and lacks the strength to perform any single worthwhile action. Learned skills may have been forgotten and movement patterns may need a certain degree of re-education. Separate movements must be practised and strengthened in such a way as to lead to strong intrinsic movements of the hand and full function. A list of suggested uses of Theraplast which will help in this final important stage of rehabilitation is given below. At first the Theraplast should be well moulded by the physiotherapist before it is offered to the patient. Soon he will do this chore for himself.

Strengthening of hand movements in the final stages of rehabilitation.

1. *Wrist extension* (with the ability to hold the position of the full recovery pattern, as in Figure 73a, against mild manual resistance).

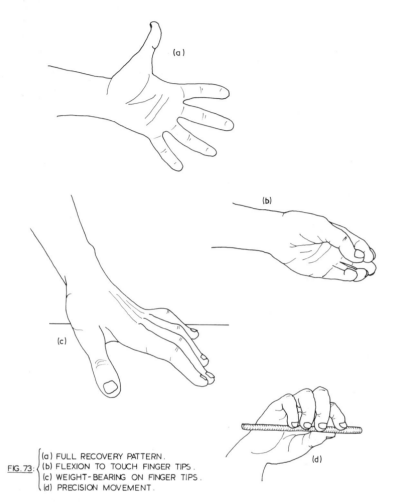

FIG. 73:
(a) FULL RECOVERY PATTERN.
(b) FLEXION TO TOUCH FINGER TIPS.
(c) WEIGHT-BEARING ON FINGER TIPS.
(d) PRECISION MOVEMENT.

(a) The hands are pressed together in an attitude of prayer with thumbs and fingers abducted and a piece of Theraplast is held firmly between the heels of the hands and the palms. Wrist extension is practised, first as a passive movement with the assistance of the sound hand and then as a graduated active/resisted movement working against the sound hand. Elbows should be firmly supported on a table.

(b) Roll out a piece of Theraplast, pressing down on the palm and keeping the fingers extended when pushing away and straight when pulling back. Here, again, use Plasticine.

(c) Flatten a piece of Theraplast and place the hand firmly onto it, palm down and fingers extended and abducted. Lift the hand off the

Theraplast by extending the wrist but leave the heel of the hand in contact.

2. *Wrist flexion*

(a) The hands are positioned as in (a) above. Wrist flexion is practised using the sound hand to give graduated resistance to the affected hand.

(b) The hand is positioned as in (c) above. Wrist flexion is practised by lifting the palm of the hand away from the Theraplast and leaving the fingers in contact.

3. *Combined wrist movements*

Wring out a handful of Theraplast.

4. *Finger flexion/extension* (or grip/release).

Grip a lump of Theraplast firmly to give a deep imprint, then release, opening the hand to extend the fingers.

5. *Finger extension*

(a) Make a Theraplast doughnut large enough to enclose the fingers and thumb as in Figure 73b. Push open the doughnut by extending the fingers and thumb.

(b) Place the hand flat down on a piece of Theraplast with fingers and thumb extended and abducted as in Exercise 1(c) above. Press the hand firmly into place and then pull it backwards through the theraplast.

6. *Opposition*

(a) Pinch and pull out small pieces of Theraplast from a lump held in the sound hand, using thumb and first finger, thumb and second finger, and so on.

(b) Make pinch marks along the top of a strip of Theraplast that has been rolled to suitable thickness and pressed firmly onto the table.

(c) Weight-bear on the finger-tips, as in Figure 73c, on a flattened piece of Theraplast and pull the fingers and thumb backwards into opposition.

(d) Roll a very small piece of Theraplast between thumb and fingers.

7. *Weight-bearing* on the finger-tips.

Stand up and place the finger-tips (as in Fig. 73c) on a *thick* flattened wedge of Theraplast. Press thumb and finger-tips firmly into the Theraplast and practise supporting an increasing amount of weight over controlled finger-tips.

The physiotherapist who is new to Theraplast ought to try out these suggested exercises herself and get the feel of using the material before she gives it to her patient. It has many possibilities and she will find it to be an extremely valuable rehabilitation aid. The depth of the imprint her patient makes on the material will indicate his strength or his weakness, and this will help her to assess his muscle power accurately and so to devise suitable therapeutic exercises. Plasticine will also prove a useful aid towards rehabilitation of small precision movements. Theraplast must be kept in a container when not in use or it spreads. Plasticine can be moulded into any desired shape and left to harden. Figure 73d illustrates delicate precision handling of a rod made from Plasticine. Such a rod could not be made from Theraplast and left to harden. It would simply spread. This is the only advantage Plasticine has over Theraplast. I use both Theraplast and plasticine. It is best to keep an open mind and flexible treatment plans which will be arranged to suit the needs of the individual patient. The only rigid necessity is that the physiotherapist should keep within the bounds laid down by a clear understanding of the principles behind all successful rehabilitation of stroke patients.

Small balls of Plasticine and lumps of sorbo rubber or plastic foam of various sizes also make good handling objects for precision movements. Controlled and delicate finger-tip pressure may be used. Span, spherical, cylindrical, key and pinch grips should all be used.

For full rehabilitation, it is frequently necessary to include practice in carrying out a sequence of movements, or a series of actions, which the patient repeats under supervision and memorises for 'homework'. This is essential where retraining of forgotten skills is undertaken. It is best to start with a simple sequence and to make full use of vision, touch and hearing. For example, I sometimes use a little red leather dog filled with sand which was given to me by a patient who found it to be a most useful aid to recovery. The leather is brightly coloured, pliable and conforms readily to the shape of the cupped hand giving sensory stimulation by vision and touch. Movement commands are given slowly and clearly. An example of a simple sequence of movements is given below.

The patient sits at the table leaning on parallel forearms, palms down. The dog is placed on the table to the right of the right hand. The sequence of movement goes from right to left.
Commands:
'Pick up the dog with your left hand.'
'Place your left arm back on the table.'
'Transfer the dog to your right hand.'
'Place your left hand back on the table.'
'Put the dog down on your left-hand side.'
'Place your right hand back on the table.'
Repeat the sequence moving from left to right. If the commands do not gain the required response, demonstrate the exercise. Assist the patient to learn the sequence by repetition and when it is thoroughly mastered see if it is remembered on the following day. The ability to memorise and carry out a series of actions will be used in assessment. In cases of impaired mental alertness this hand rehabilitation exercise would not be given. *Note:* It must be remembered that assessment tests ought not to be used as routine rehabilitation exercises.

On the same lines, 'pat-a-cake' may be used. This is the simple 'game' where the physiotherapist and the patient sit facing each other and clap hands in an arranged sequence; for example, they clap their own hands once, then clap right hand to right hand, clap their own hands again, then clap left hand to left hand, clap their own hands, clap both hands to both hands . . . and so on. They sit facing each other across a narrow table and lean on their elbows. No chance must be given for a return to any part of the spasm pattern. Again note that this is one of the 'games' used to amuse a small child and develops concentration and coordination. For this reason, care must be taken that 'pat-a-cake' will not be used where it is likely to offend the patient's ego.

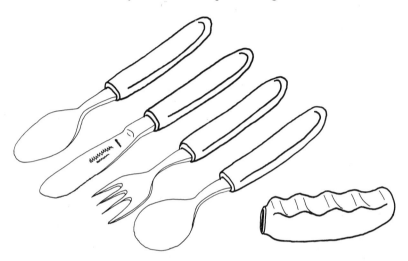

FIG. 74: SELECTAGRIP CUTLERY.

Figure 74: Selectagrip Cutlery may be brought into use to advantage *when* the patient reaches an advanced enough stage to begin using both hands for feeding. Various sizes of grip are available. The handgrip slides over the handle of the implement and as soon as the largest grip has been mastered it may be removed and a smaller one substituted. It may be useful to know that Polyform, a low temperature othotic plastic material designed specifically for the therapist, also offers an ideal material to be used to adapt equipment to suit the patient's handgrip at this stage.

Figure 75: The bath mat for table use is a helpful idea where the friction-free polished surface of the table does not allow the patient to support himself over his forearms. A bath mat cut in half will supply two patients with this necessary extra aid and gives a very suitable non-shifting surface for forearm support in all table activities right through the rehabilitation programme. It is always necessary to see that the patient's chair is high enough to allow him to lean forward over the table and so over his forearms.

In the final stages of hand rehabilitation, an electric vibrator—which

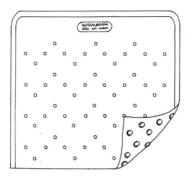

FIG.75: BATH MAT FOR TABLE USE.

the lay person may buy in any chemist, to be used for mechanical massage—perhaps has a part to play. I sometimes use one. Again, it was supplied by an anxious patient who had his family bring it into hospital because he thought it would help his hand. He was convinced it did.

Figure 76: An example of writing restored, was done by the right-sided stroke patient who found the red leather dog so helpful and later presented it to me. Six weeks before he wrote this page his morale was at a very low ebb because he couldn't even sign a cheque. He had motor and sensory (proprioceptive) loss and was treated with pressure splints, both with intermittent and sustained pressure, and the full course of arm

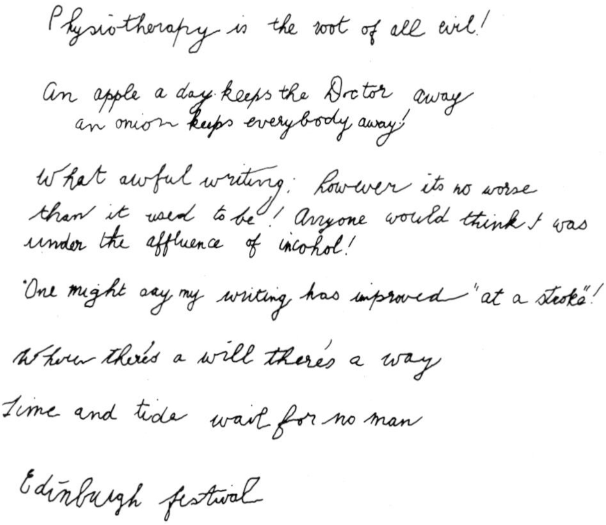

Physiotherapy is the root of all evil!

An apple a day keeps the Doctor away
an onion keeps everybody away!

What awful writing. However its no worse
than it used to be! Anyone would think I was
under the affluence of incohol!

One might say my writing has improved "at a stroke"!

Where there's a will there's a way

Time and tide wait for no man

Edinburgh festival

FIG.76 : AN EXAMPLE OF WRITING RESTORED.

rehabilitation as suggested here. He also insisted on trying the electric vibrator on the palm of his hand and said it made the 'dead' area deep between his metacarpals feel 'alive'. We also used music therapy and he began 'playing the drums' on a table top with free left-hand movement and a very wooden right hand until one day he got very excited because he had 'got his rhythm back'. He was playing the drums with equally relaxed hands. He had been a competent pianist. He refused to make any attempt at playing the piano until he himself was satisfied he was ready to make a successful attempt with something like his former skill. A month after he gave me this example of writing restored he began playing the piano again. It would have been impossible to tell that he had had a fairly severe stroke. He was in his late seventies. It will be seen that he had a sense of humour—one of the greatest aids in all stroke rehabilitation.

Note: Elbow support for hand activities is maintained until the patient is ready to begin rhythm sessions.

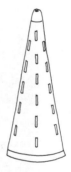

FIG. 77: WOOLLEN CONE

Figure 77: A cone from the woollen mill gives an example of an article that is most useful in hand rehabilitation. On the look out for new ideas, I came across a box full of these cones recently. They fit one inside the other. With one fastened securely to a board to make a suitable base, they may be used for stacking and unstacking. They may be set out in suitable positions and the sequence for picking up may be varied. Their shape encourages a grip with very good opposition of the thumb. Many people try to put the cart before the horse. It is unrealistic, frustrating and even demoralising if an attempt to fasten buttons is demanded before wrist and finger control has been established.

Figure 78 shows the ideal shape for an orally inflatable pressure splint for the arm. It does not taper towards the hand and allows ample room to spread the fingers and thumb in wide abduction. The long inflating tube with the detachable mouthpiece is both hygienic and practical in

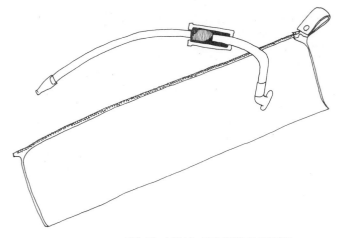

FIG. 78: URIAS PRESSURE SPLINT

use, as is the easily closed clip off valve. It should be applied as previously described with the arm in the complete anti-spasm or recovery pattern and it should be inflated to full lung pressure. This latest design in orally inflatable splints has only come into my possession for the first time in recent weeks and I find it most satisfactory for the reasons given above. It is marketed by *Urias* of Denmark. On the other hand, the United States splint as described earlier, is more pliable and exercise routines are more easily performed, particularly where the splint is used to give the stability of sustained posture while weight is applied from the heel of the hand to the externally rotated shoulder. Full wrist extension is more easily obtained in the U.S. splint. The broader zip on the Urias splint might give uncushioned pressure if the splint is not very carefully applied. Make sure to position the finger-tips well back from the open end of all pressure splints and position the zip as shown in Figure 30.

Note: It is to be hoped that a manufacturer will shortly produce the ideal splint which combines the best features of both.

Figure 79 shows the final satisfaction, as seen by the artist, of the stroke victim who has been rehabilitated and is ready to face normal living. He walks with balanced, correct gait and is proud of his useful arm, used here to carry his hat. Until this final result is obtained, if we are dealing with the complete stroke and our aim is full rehabilitation, each treatment must have a progressive approach. But, at the same time, even if it means going back in the treatment programme, any difficulty that is encountered must be faced and mastered. The skill of the physiotherapist must be used to obtain the desired result. She must lead her patient through treatment sessions which he enjoys and which are satisfactory because he gains confidence from her approach and the sure

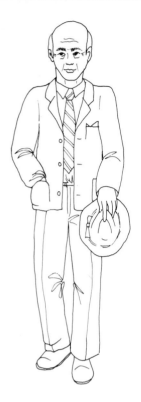

FIG. 79: SATISFACTION

knowledge that he is making progress. It must never be forgotten by the physiotherapist that her patient has suffered severe mental as well as physical trauma. She must help him to rehabilitate his mind as well as his body. His ego has been subjected to a stupefying blow.

Methods used to stimulate and reinforce underlying postural mechanisms will continue to be used right through the programme and, in the case of arm rehabilitation, I find the use of orally inflatable pressure splints is always necessary. It supplies the missing stability of sustained posture that is necessary for rehabilitation. Approximation from the heel of the hand through an extended elbow to an externally rotated shoulder plays a vital part in successful treatment and should continue to be given—*with and without the aid of a pressure splint*—as part of each treatment session all the way through the final stages of hand rehabilitation. The importance of weight-bearing on the finger-tips must not be forgotten.

To those who say I make extravagant claims for the use of pressure splints in the treatment of the stroke patient's affected arm, I would say that I can only base my findings on the consistently satisfactory results I have obtained over a period of ten years. I have not carried out independent clinical trials but I have compared the overall results I have achieved with the results many of my colleagues are obtaining elsewhere and I have found, in general, the treatment results obtained elsewhere leave much to be desired. It was in an attempt to solve the residual problem of the hemiplegic arm that I first became interested in the possibilities offered by the pressure splint. If I compare the results I have achieved by using the splint with those I achieved formerly without its use (almost without exception they were most unsatisfactory) I am left in no doubt about the necessary part these splints must play in a large number of cases if there is to be any hope of satisfactory rehabilitation. I would again point out that they must be applied correctly and, while in position, the exercise routines suggested here are a necessary part of treatment. To omit the exercise is to gain a poor response.

Physiotherapists must continue to look for new ideas and pool their findings. Successful stroke treatment and the prevention of residual disability must be our aim. We may not achieve this in every case but there is no reason why we should not with many. With deficit in proprioceptive sense and the consequent failure of anti-gravity and postural mechanisms, we have been faced with the greatest hurdle blocking the way to recovery. With the help of the pressure splint and a carefully planned programme of exercises I have found a way round this hurdle. These patients need no longer be faced with severe and persistent handicap and no hope of recovery; we can, and we must, substantially increase the numbers in the recovery group who go back to a useful life. Then we can say: 'We are good enough.'

Conclusions

Successful rehabilitation, as presented here, depends on the physiotherapist and her ability to understand the basic principles of treatment and to interpret these principles into a sound and realistic physical programme which will facilitate controlled movement and recovery. She must keep an open mind, *make a cheerful and hopeful approach,* and she must find ways and means of getting round other difficulties that are likely to be present in the elderly patient—e.g. the heart condition, vascular complications, arthritis of the knee, respiratory insufficiency, the old fracture that was set in the spasm pattern. The conclusions reached show that the physiotherapist must:

1. Re-establish the postural reflex mechanism by using the spinal reflex arc and working upwards.

2. Use positioning at all times to inhibit dominating reflexes.

3. Recognise sensory loss where present and use every method in the book (or find new ones) to step up sensory input.

4. Assess the tonal pattern correctly and use the appropriate methods to inhibit or reinforce according to the findings.

5. Understand why all patients, whatever the tonal pattern, lose the

ability to place and hold the affected limb in space.

6. Establish proximal to distal movement control.

7. Understand the principles behind the need for lateral transference of weight over the affected side.

8. Understand the principles behind reinforcement of postural mechanisms in weight-bearing.

9. Understand the need for meticulous positioning of the base in weight-bearing (this must include point 10).

10. Understand the need to weight-bear over a correctly positioned hand.

11. Establish the final sequence of distal to proximal movement.

5. Assessment

General assessment

I have left until last the chapter which many physiotherapists might prefer to find at the beginning. I have done this deliberately because I do not believe it is possible to make reliable stroke assessments without a sound working knowledge of the principles behind stroke rehabilitation. In particular, the difficulties that may be encountered in the parietal lobe syndrome are more ably approached and better understood if they are approached with this sound working knowledge. Rehabilitation methods do not change—application may be more difficult and the physiotherapist will be called on to use all her skill and ingenuity to meet the patient's needs. Without experience it is impossible to begin to understand or to make a realistic approach to the complicated problems that may be found on careful assessment—and *experience is necessary before reliable assessment is possible.*

Very careful assessment is necessary so that the particular problem of each patient may be diagnosed, understood, and approached in a positive way. The problems may include motor loss and/or sensory loss and the consequent problems of sensorimotor function and perceptual difficulties. But there are other problems. These may include problems of intellectual function, problems of communication, psychological problems, family problems, employment problems and social problems. It is a daunting list but this only makes it all the more urgently necessary to unearth the difficulties that may stand in the way of recovery and a return to normal living. It must be remembered, for example, that a breakdown in a marriage relationship that has led to many years of unhappy acceptance of an unsatisfactory way of life can, after the onset of a stroke, completely block the necessary hopeful approach to rehabilitation that must be made by the patient himself if success is to be achieved.

Primarily, it is the business of the physiotherapist to understand and deal with the problems of disfunction involving sensorimotor disturbance. Her approach to rehabilitation may be said to be a sensorimotor approach. In making this sensorimotor approach and setting down a broad plan of treatment, by and large I have dealt with the methods I use to approach these problems. But it is also necessary to have a full understanding of exactly what is meant by saying the patient will be faced with sensorimotor problems. I have advanced and discussed a method that may be most effectively used to step up sensory input to the limb that demonstrates sensory loss but, where sensory loss is at a high functional level, we become involved in the many difficulties which may be included in the parietal lobe syndrome and the problems presented may often seem indissoluble. These problems may include any of the following difficulties.

1. Loss of proprioceptive sense which leads to *disturbances in body image,* body image being the ability to feel a limb, to appreciate the movements of the joints and to appreciate its place in space and its relationship to the body. Many patients have difficulties which present as *agnosia* (difficulty in recognition) and this may go as far as neglect or denial of ownership (*anosognosia*) or may even include denial of paralysis. As I have already said, proprioceptive sense automatically controls anti-gravity and postural mechanisms and, without this control, resulting severe handicap poses an enormous problem, the stability of sustained posture being essential for purposeful movement.

2. Impairment of tactile sensation with impairment of ability to recognise objects placed in the hand (*astereognosis*) and impairment of coordination of sensory input which gives *disturbance of spatial relationships.* If the brain is no longer aware of body image the patient will be incapable of determining his position in space.

(Sensory messages from proprioceptors of muscles and joints, from proprioceptors of the neck in response to movement of the head, and changes in muscle tone by stimulation of the labyrinths, all contribute to the brain's awareness of body image—or brain awareness of the different parts of the body and their relationship to space.)

3. *Apraxic problems* which result from a disturbance of visuo-spatial orientation, or, because of the disorder of body image, lead to inability to deal effectively with or manipulate objects e.g. *dressing apraxia.*

4. Problems in carrying out voluntary actions using objects in the environment (or space), or inability to copy designs of more than one dimension usually recognised as *constructional apraxia.*

5. Problems of *left-right discrimination.*

6. Disturbances in *visual perception* which may include the ability to distinguish between vertical and horizontal positioning of an object held up in space. This is *visual agnosia* which must be recognised as a perceptual difficulty and not as blindness. The patient can see the object but he cannot assess its position in relationship to his own body image. If visual agnosia is present in a bilateral lesion the effect is devastating. In unilateral lesions compensation may be made. The patient who keeps bumping into objects and misjudging distances ought to be tested for visual agnosia. (Hemianopia is a quite different condition and does concern blindness of half of the visual field.)

Note on apraxic problems: These problems are often found to be present where there is no severe paralysis and they come under two headings:

1. *Ideomotor.* Ideomotor apraxia: the patient is incapable of carrying out purposeful movement on command, or of imitating gestures, while routine, automatic activities will still be performed. For example, if brushing his teeth was a former routine action, if he is presented with his toothbrush he will brush his teeth because the action is automatic. But if he is told to polish a horse brass with the toothbrush he will fail to carry out this new idea which is not automatic.

2. *Ideational.* Ideational apraxia: the patient will fail in the automatic task. He will not brush his teeth when presented with his toothbrush.

Note: Study of the Greek derivations can help our understanding. For example there is a word *ideopraxist*, one who is impelled to carry out an idea, from the Greek *idea*, idea and *praxis*, doing.

An understanding of these problems is essential if an intelligent approach is to be made to rehabilitation. With understanding, ideomotor disability may often be turned into successful movement. The patient may fail completely if he is given supporting assistance in standing and asked to concentrate on his leg movement and walk. But, if a cup of coffee is placed on a table on the other side of the room and he is told: 'There is your coffee. Go and get it!' he will often step out and cross the room.

Where sensorimotor disturbances are present it is an established fact that, where the non-dominant hemisphere is involved, the difficulties are greater than those found where the dominant hemisphere is involved *but* this does not apply to the area concerned with left-right discrimination. This means the lesions of the dominant hemisphere have greater difficulty with left-right discrimination and, added to this, they may also present bilateral apraxic problems.

It can be seen, then, how important careful assessment is but there is one more point that the physiotherapist must take into account. Performance with the stroke patient may vary considerably from day to day and a hasty assessment will tend to be unreliable. Careful and thorough assessment is the business of the occupational therapist and, where necessary, the skill of the speech therapist ought to be included. For most of us it is impossible to imagine how the brain can produce the whole complex world of our perception and it takes a fairly highly trained person to assess intellectual and cognitive problems thoroughly, particularly where language disorder further complicates the issue. But, if an intelligent and realistic approach to rehabilitation is to be made by the physiotherapist, she must understand the few simple tests that will give her an overall picture of the problems involved. How else can she make an intelligent approach to rehabilitation? Also, a reliable assessment cannot be made immediately after the onset of the stroke. It will take time. *And it is very wrong to make an early arbitrary assessment on prognosis.* It will be a full month after onset before a prognosis assessment of motor involvement (with no sensory involvement) may be in any way reliable. Where sensory involvement is also included the time necessary to reach a reliable prognosis assessment will be twice as long and, if there is parietal lobe syndrome included, the prognosis assessment time will be three to four months. *And* these figures depend on intensive physiotherapy and correct handling. *And* the correct plan to be followed in the intensive physiotherapy programme depends on *regular and careful progress assessment.* So it must be realised that *treatment assessment* and *prognosis assessment* are not one and the same thing. From the very early days the physiotherapist must be able to make reliable treatment assessments and this will include the state of muscle tone, motor loss, sensory loss and parietal lobe involvement.

The physiotherapist must be able to assess:

1. *The state of muscle tone.* Practice will lead to reliable efficiency and she will be able to assess spasticity, flaccidity and intension tremor or a co-existence of all three. At its simplest level, she will do this if she moves the affected limb passively fully into the recovery pattern. If the limb is in any way resistant to the passive movement, spasticity is present. If, on the other hand, the limb is not resistant but it is heavy and abnormally relaxed it is lacking in tone, or flaccid. Where severe, abnormally flaccid muscles are found, sensory tests ought to be carried out with very special care.

Some degree of spasticity is almost always present in the stroke patient. Even if the arm seems to be completely flaccid, it usually demonstrates flexor spasm in the fingers when strong stretch is applied and held and mild resistance to full passive movement of the shoulder will be found. Similarly, if the leg seems to be completely flaccid, passive flexion of the hip and knee meet with mild resistance when the patient lies supine.

Note: It will be remembered that this accurate assessment is vital because there are always changes in normal muscle tone in stroke patients and, according to her findings, the physiotherapist will take the appropriate measures to restore tone.

2. *Motor loss.* Motor loss means loss of controlled movement. The success or failure of the whole rehabilitation plan may depend on the physiotherapist's ability to estimate motor loss correctly. It must by now be quite obvious that it is not only bad practice but positively harmful to recovery if the patient is asked to weight-bear on a limb that has not got controlled movement of the proximal joint—i.e. hip or shoulder. Controlled movement must be re-educated in the hip and shoulder before it can be expected to be present in the knee and elbow. And controlled movement in the knee and elbow, either actively or with assistance, ought to be present if weight-bearing over a correctly positioned foot or hand is to lead to distal control and development of controlled movement from distal to proximal.

Gross motor patterns will be used initially to test for controlled hip and shoulder movement, remembering that rolling may be used as a mass flexion or a mass extension pattern. The patient who has not learnt to roll and is quite unable to roll from supine to prone, or prone to supine leading with the affected side will be found to be deficient in hip and/or shoulder control. Controlled knee movement may be assessed (where hip control has been established) with the patient in side-lying on the affected side, or in supine lying by assisted active movement and the ability to hold the limb in space. Controlled elbow movement will be tested with the limb placed fully in the recovery pattern. Assessment results will indicate the stage reached in the rehabilitation plan and careful motor assessment at regular intervals will give a suitable yardstick on which to base a progress report.

3. *Sensory loss.* Again, to assess sensory loss quickly and easily the physiotherapist usually makes a beginning by using a few simple tests which are easily carried out. Loss of *proprioception* is tested by passive movements of the index finger and big toe. The patient watches the movement. Then his eyes are covered and he is asked to say if each movement is 'up' or 'down'. If he is uncertain, or he does not know, the larger joints are tested. Or, with his eyes blindfolded, the physiotherapist may move his affected arm into various positions and he will be asked to repeat the movement with his sound arm. Or, first using his eyes and then blindfolded, he is asked to grasp the thumb of the affected hand while the physiotherapist changes the thumb's position. *Sensation* must also be tested. Cutaneous sensibility, or tactile sensation, must be assessed by asking the blindfolded patient to identify light touch on any part of his body. Two point discrimination is also used, the result of the test depending on the patient's ability to distinguish two points from one on the finger pulps without using eyesight. Or tests in *stereognosis* may fail. These are tests where objects held in the hand are recognised by touch without using eyesight. Some people use familiar objects—such as a key, a comb, a coin or a ball—and ask for identification of the object. Others use shapes of different kinds and texture and ask for identification of shape, size and texture. One of the problems with this test is that the patient must be able to move the object, or at least move fingers over it, in order to recognise it; with motor loss this is impossible and therefore I find it a not altogether satisfactory test in the stroke patient. Where sensory loss of any kind is found to be present every effort must be made to step up sensory input. It perhaps ought to be pointed out that, as well as having a positive effect on proprioceptive loss, pressure splints also have a positive effect on cutaneous receptors—particularly on the palms of the hands and the soles of the feet where large numbers of receptors have specific sensitivity to pressure.

4. *Parietal lobe involvement.* If the meaning of parietal lobe involvement is understood, assessment becomes easier—or relatively less difficult. For assessment purposes, it is probably helpful to divide the lobes under two headings, dominant and non-dominant.

Where *the dominant lobe* is involved any of the following disabilities may be present.

(a) Bilateral apraxia—(ideomotor) as already described.

(b) Tactile astereognosis—as above.

(c) Postural difficulties—which may show as a lateral lean.

(d) Right/left disorientation: difficulty in identifying right/left.

(e) Finger agnosia: the patient has difficulty in identifying his fingers.

(f) Dysgraphia: difficulty in writing.

(g) Dyscalculia: difficulty in simple mental arithmetic and adding.

Remember to make allowance for any pre-stroke difficulty.

Where *the non-dominant lobe* is involved we may look for some similar disabilities and some a little different.

(a) Constructional apraxia

(b) Tactile astereognosis

(c) Postural difficulties

(d) Disorder of spatial judgment

(e) Visual agnosia

(f) Anosognosia—neglect or denial of ownership of the affected limbs

(g) Disturbance of body image.

Obviously where there is parietal lobe involvement, or where it is necessary to exclude parietal lobe involvement, careful assessment must be made and this is where the skilled occupational therapist can be a tremendous help. But she may not always be available and, in any case, it is necessary for the physiotherapist to understand some of the simpler tests and, for treatment planning and progress reporting, she must be able to make simple assessments.

Under the heading of general assessment I have already discussed some of the problems encountered. When considering quick assessment for parietal lobe involvement, it must be remembered performance may vary considerably from day to day.

Draw an arrow is a test that may be used as a quick way of identifying brain damage which, if demonstrated by this test, will possibly be in the parietal lobe area. The patient is asked to draw an arrow on a clean sheet of paper. If it is poorly formed, misshapen or the point inverted this is a fair indication of brain damage which is possibly indicated more substantially if the test is continued further and again fails. The patient is asked to *copy an arrow* and failure is demonstrated where repeated copying shows changing or deteriorating form.

Draw a man is another useful quick test, the response demonstrating different disabilities. In almost every case it is necessary to explain that the ability or inability to draw is not important. Where loss of body image is present body parts in the drawing will be missing, wrongly placed or indistinguishable. The patient's performance is watched carefully as it gives an indication of underlying disability. He may make all sorts of excuses to avoid the test and gentle persuasion may be needed before he sets about the task.

Performance		Possible Interpretation
Repetitive scribbling	=	Perseveration
Body parts missing and/or disrupted	=	Agnosia and disturbance of body image
Failure to draw coherently	=	Apraxia
Omission of left half of the drawing	=	Neglect of left half of space
Drawing positioned on the right half of the page	=	Neglect of left half of space
Very small drawing	=	Tendency to dementia

Draw a clock is another favourite test used to assess parietal lobe involvement. Again the physiotherapist must watch the patient's performance with great care and make her assessment. For example:

Performance		Interpretation
Repeated drawing of circles	=	Perseveration
Drawing of circle with left half missing	=	Neglect of left half of space
Numbers not all within the circle	=	General brain damage
Numbers on the left side omitted	=	Neglect of left half of space

Draw a house is the third drawing demand I frequently make.

Performance		Interpretation
Misplaced windows, doors, or chimneys	=	Agnosia
Minimal or no detail and no perspective	=	Possible not high intellect prior to stroke, or brain damage

And so on. Practice in assessment leads to correct interpretation of the drawing produced. A list of points to be watched for and to be noted when the patient responds to the demand to draw will be given below.

Copying drawings can be useful to test for apraxia, disorder of spatial judgment and anosognosia (neglect or denial of ownership of the affected limbs). The same three subjects—a man, a clock and a house—are usually used again. Remember that each new drawing is done on a fresh piece of paper and one drawing is completed (within the patient's capability) before the next is attempted. Allowance will be made in all of these drawing tests for the patient who is using an affected dominant hand or an unaffected non-dominant hand. A felt-tip pen is least difficult to hold. The drawings to be copied are not done beforehand. They should be done in front of the patient as a demonstration of exactly what is required of him. The physiotherapist will again watch the patient carefully and interpret his performance.

Copy a two-dimensional geometric figure (a box or a pyramid) may be included here and failure in this test will indicate two-dimensional apraxia. Or the patient may be asked to copy designs using matchsticks as a test for two-dimensional constructional apraxia.

Neglect of one half of space is very quickly demonstrated when two brightly coloured pens of contrasting colours are held in front of the patient about one foot apart and he fails to identify one of them. The patient with neglect of, say, the left half of space will only see the pen in the right visual field. *Note:* the patient with hemianopia will only see one pen *but* he will see both of the pens if they are interchanged in front of his eyes because he is able to follow the pen that moves into the blind half of his visual field. In cases of severe neglect of half of space, only one pen is seen even when they are moved so that they are in front of the patient and less than one inch apart. Even when they are interchanged in front of the patient's eyes he will not be able to follow the pen that moves into the blind half of his visual field.

Agnosia is loss of the power to perceive. Therefore it is readily understood what a devastating effect visual agnosia can have—particularly when the condition is bilateral. It means that the patient is able to see but he cannot interpret what he sees. Wherever visual agnosia is present it must be diagnosed and the finding noted down on the assessment sheet. The physiotherapist who works with stroke patients can find assessment a fascinating business provided she sets out to assess with a reasonable understanding of the difficulties she may encounter. With understanding she quickly learns to interpret the drawings that are produced.

Interpretation of drawings which should be done on separate clean sheets of paper using a felt-tipped pen.

(a) Make allowances for left-handed drawing by the right-handed patient.

(b) Always note the position of the drawing on the page, remembering that patients with neglect of the left half of space place their drawings on the right half of the page.

(c) Note the size of the drawing, remembering that demented patients tend to make a very small drawing.

(d) An elaborate detailed drawing tends to point to a high intellectual level prior to the stroke.

(e) Note the placing of the parts of the body which will be disrupted, grossly misshapen, or missing in cases of agnosia.

(f) Leaving out the left half of a drawing—e.g. a house—indicates visual agnosia, or severe neglect of the left half of space.

(g) Incoherent drawing will indicate receptive dysphasia or apraxia, repetitive scribbling should be noted as evidence of perseveration.

(h) The drawing with a lateral lean, or the progressive lateral lean of repeated arrows may indicate postural difficulties.

(i) The clock with numbers wandering outside the face indicates general brain damage—as distinct from the clock with numbers omitted in cases of spatial neglect.

Before leaving parietal lobe involvement it might be helpful to make two more observations.

Strike a match may be used as a quick test for apraxia where motor function is present. The patient is simply given a box of matches and asked to strike a match while his performance is watched and noted.

Gerstmann's syndrome may occur where the dominant parietal lobe is involved and demonstrates as (a) difficulty with writing, (b) difficulty with number calculation, (c) right and left disorientation and (d) finger agnosia. *Note:* Many people suffer from a touch of Gerstmann's syndrome—difficulty with mental arithmetic for example—and probably the physiotherapist need not probe into any difficulty associated with Gerstmann's syndrome but she ought to understand what it means. This may include the following tests.

1. *Dysgraphia* will be detected if the patient is asked to write down a simple sentence which is dictated by the tester, e.g. 'Tomorrow is Saturday', and he fails.

2. *Dyscalculia* will be detected if the patient fails to do simple mental arithmetic or to add up three columns of figures.

3. *Right and left disorientation* will be detected if the patient is unable to identify his own right and left hands followed by identifying the tester's right and left hands when she sits opposite him with her hands crossed.

4. *Finger agnosia* will be detected if the patient is unable to identify his own fingers on his affected hand and on his unaffected hand and the fingers on the tester's hand.

The physiotherapist's assessment, then, must include these points:

1. *The state of muscle tone*
2. *Motor loss*
3. *Sensory loss*
4. *Parietal lobe involvement.*

But there still remains two other possible deficits which must be considered for complete assessment.

5. *Hearing loss* and
6. *Visual loss* which has been touched on very briefly above.

5. *Hearing loss,* where present, must be recognised in the early days. It may be due to auditory agnosia. As in visual agnosia, the function is present but cannot be interpreted. The necessary simple examination to exclude wax or a non-functioning hearing aid as the cause of deafness will be made before a more complex diagnosis is sought. The physician will assess the damage. Deafness may result from trouble in the middle ear, the inner ear, or from damage to nerve or brain stem, or as a result of receptive dysphasia and impaired comprehension.

Whatever the cause, the important factor from the physiotherapist's point of view, is to recognise the deficit where it is present and to treat the patient accordingly.

For efficient and kindly treatment the physiotherapist must understand the following facts:

(a) Patients must not be shouted at, particularly where there is a perceptual deficit which gives distorted hearing and the patient cannot tolerate noise.

(b) Instructions should be simple and manual contact and mime must be used to gain the required response during treatment sessions.

(c) Depression is common after the onset of a stroke, particularly where hearing loss is present. This may show as withdrawal and unhappy isolation.

(d) The condition may vary from day to day, the patient showing improvement when morale is high. This results from the confidence gained by efficient rehabilitation.

(e) The deficit frequently resolves in the first month or two after the onset of the stroke but, for the reason given above, it must not be missed during the early assessment.

6. *Visual loss* has been discussed above where it presents as a perceptive deficit and it has been pointed out that visual agnosia (the patient can see but cannot interpret what he sees) must not be confused with hemianopia. Hemianopia is blindness (the patient cannot see) in one half of the visual field, of one or both eyes. A test for hemianopia has been suggested but the simplest and quickest test is made by approaching the patient waving two brightly coloured flowers simultaneously from both sides of his visual field. He will ignore the flower in the blind half of the field. Or, if the physiotherapist makes simultaneous finger movements bilaterally in both sides of the visual field, the movement will be picked up on the unaffected side and ignored on the affected side. Improvement can be expected and the patient who is aware of the deficit is easily taught to rotate his head to compensate for the hopefully temporary disability. His rehabilitation programme depends on frequent and persistent rotation into rolling as already described and, for this reason, it does not make sense to suggest that his locker ought to be placed on his sighted side. He must be encouraged to rotate across the affected side if rehabilitation is to be successful. Note that this may be particularly necessary for successful rehabilitation where the right non-dominant lobe is affected because the patient may be unaware of the visual defect and also of the left disability (anosognosia). Manual contacts will play a considerable part in physical rehabilitation to establish the rolling routines necessary to reach for the locker, to roll to sitting, to roll to sitting to getting out of bed and in all the early physiotherapy routines. Those who attend the patient will greatly assist his progress if they approach him from his affected side and assist him into a suitable rolling position for communication. Rolling to elbow propping ought to be established quickly.

Conclusion on rehabilitation to be given for the patient with perceptual loss. The whole line of thought that has been presented in this book and followed throughout the rehabilitation programme again makes sound sense and often obtains surprisingly satisfactory results where perceptual difficulty is encountered. Re-education of body awareness, visuo-spatial orientation and object recognition depend on normal integration of impulses from the cerebral cortical areas concerned with vision, hearing, cutaneous sensibility and proprioception. Sensory messages from the proprioceptors of muscles and joints, from proprioceptors of the neck (with head movements) and changes in muscle tone by stimulation of the labyrinths all contribute to the brain's awareness of the body scheme and visuo-spatial orientation. Therefore, where there is deficit in body awareness, visuo-spatial orientation and object recognition it makes sound sense to step up the afferent impulses by way of the fullest possible stimulation of proprioceptors—using superficial and deep pressure, rolling and approximation to bombard the proprioceptors—alerting every available afferent impulse to assist in re-establishing the necessary degree of integration of impulses at cortical level to obtain normal function.

It must be fairly obvious by now that it makes nonsense of this whole approach to stroke rehabilitation if we insist that testing for the identification of perceptual disability in the stroke patient is wholly the business of the occupational therapist. If she is to make an intelligent approach to her patient's needs, the physiotherapist must have a few necessary simple tests at her finger-tips and she must be able to make a reasonable assessment. Where she finds perceptual and cognitive disturbance to be present she will, if she is lucky, be able to call on the skill of the highly trained occupational therapist who ought to be able to come up with a complete picture of the patient's difficulty. Where necessary, occupational and speech therapists will combine on assessment and, e.g., high level receptive difficulty will not be missed.

I believe that the physiotherapist who works with stroke patients must be proficient in testing, she must not forget to take into account any visual or auditory impairment and she must be well up in her subject. She ought to read anything the experts have to offer. Each physiotherapist will tend to adopt her own favourite tests that are carried out without any stress or frustration for her patient and, with careful explanation and handling, she will not be faced by the angry patient who is not prepared to play 'children's games'. I compiled my first list of tests from the book I earlier recommended to physiotherapists— *Cerebrovascular Disability* by G.F. Adams, and I keep adding to the list. This gives variety and all tests are not necessarily used to assess one patient. I have among my 'box of tricks', a set of Merit Build-up Beakers and a Merit Posting Box. The beakers consist of a set of twelve beakers of diminishing size which may be built with or nested and are used to test for learning ability, abstract thinking, flexibility, apraxia and agnosia. The posting box has six holes of different shapes and six shapes which fit exactly, each through its own hole and no other. This test uncovers any difficulty with spatial comprehension, neglect of half of space and problem solving behaviour. The T shape generally seems to give most trouble and the patient's approach to the problem of finding a way to solve the posting of the various shapes ought to be noted.

As I have said, each physiotherapist will tend to adopt her own favourite tests.

Picture identification (to test for visual agnosia, neglect of left half of space and abstract thought) as demonstrated by Professor Isaacs, has become one of my favourite tests. It is quick and easy to carry out and uncovers difficulties in a minute. A picture of a man and a woman is all that is needed, preferably a bride and groom and the picture should be mounted for easy handling. The patient is shown the picture and he is asked a series of questions.

'What do you see?'

If he cannot identify the picture he is asked:

'Is there a man in it?'

'Point to the man.'

'Is there anyone else?'

'Is there a woman?'

'Point to the woman.'

'What is the woman wearing?' . . . and so on.

Interpretation of the test:

(a) Patients with *visual agnosia* fail completely.

(b) Patients with *neglect of left half of space* fail to identify figures in left half of the picture.

(c) Patients with *loss of abstract thought* fail to give a general interpretation of the picture, e.g. they call the bride a 'woman' or misidentify the picture because they misinterpret a fundamental detail, e.g. the bride is described as a nurse.

Object identification is another quick test 'borrowed' from Professor Isaacs. It can be very helpful and has become another of my favourites. It is used to test for visual agnosia, perception of colour, size, texture, function, and to detect language disturbance, especially difficulty with name-finding, also tactile agnosia (astereognosis). *Note:* this is not the blindfolded object identification test quoted above under sensory loss; it is a test which uses sight and would not be given to the blind or aphasic patient. The examiner collects a number of common objects found in the ward, making sure there is variety in colour, size and texture and including something edible, e.g. an orange. The objects are presented to the patient and he is asked to identify them. Again a series of questions will be asked about each object.

'What is this?'

'What colour is it?'

'What do you do with it?'

'Show me what you do with it.'

If the patient fails to identify an object, e.g. a sponge, it is put down in front of him beside a second very different object, e.g. a book, then more than one dissimilar object may be added and the questions asked will only apply to the sponge.

'Pick up the sponge.'
'Pick up the one with holes in it.'
'Pick up the big one.'
'Pick up the soft one.'
'Pick up the one you use to wash your face.' . . . and so on.

Where colour perception is tested and fails it may be that the patient was colour blind prior to his stroke.

Interpretation of the test:

(a) Patients with *word finding difficulty* will know the function and properties of an object while they are unable to name it.

(b) Patients with *visual agnosia* show loss of awareness of the function of objects.

(c) Patients with *tactile agnosia* show loss of ability to identify by touch.

There are many possible tests, all would not be given to any one patient but all areas of disability ought to be covered by the tests that are given to any one patient. From the physiotherapist's point of view it becomes increasingly obvious that a comprehensive assessment sheet is a necessity.

The assessment sheet

A stroke assessment sheet ought to be used and yet it remains one of the most difficult treatment aids to produce. It *is* a treatment aid because treatment will not make a balanced all-purpose approach towards the problem of rehabilitating a whole person without careful and correct assessment. Assessment sheets tend to be too brief and do not give an overall picture, or they tend to be too long (sometimes many pages) and it is impossible to see the state of the patient at a glance. It is necessary to make an attempt to draw up an assessment sheet which not only gives a clear picture of the patient's motor and sensory disability but also acts as a progress report.

Figures 80–81 give a suggested lay out for an assessment sheet which may be printed on two sides of one sheet of card. It is by no means the perfect assessment sheet but it is offered with the following suggestions.

1. It covers most of the necessary data.

2. Physiotherapists might be prepared to use it, assess its shortcomings and make improvements where necessary.

Points to remember when drawing up or using an assessment sheet.

1. Receptive and expressive ability cannot be assessed accurately immediately after a stroke. It may be some time before a high level receptive disability is picked up. An early assessment can only be a snap assessment and the examiner must keep an open mind.

2. The state of muscle tone will always be assessed with great care and it must be remembered that although tonal patterns fall into two main groups—decreased and increased tone—tremor may be present and all

Physiotherapy Stroke Assessment

Date:_____
Diagnosis:_____
Date of Onset:_____
Home Circumstances:_____
_____
Receptive Ability:_____
Expressive Ability:_____
Other Relevant Diagnoses:_____
_____

NAME:_____
ADDRESS:_____
_____
AGE:_____
OCCUPATION:_____
WARD/UNIT:_____

Muscle Tone: Are the limbs resistant to the following movements or are they heavy and
abnormally relaxed?

ARM movement into recovery pattern
plus elevation.
LEG movement into recovery pattern
plus full flexion.

DATE					
Arm					
Leg					

State: RESISTANT or HEAVY = SPASTIC or FLACCID.
= S 1 2 3 or F 1 2 3

EVALUATION OF ACTIVITIES AND PROGRESS REPORT

IN BED	DATE																							
Rolling																								
Bridging																								
Rolling to elbow propping																								
Rolling to sitting																								
IN PHYSIOTHERAPY																								
Rolling to prone lying																								
Prone lying with forearm support																								
Kneeling with forearm support																								
Full kneeling to stand kneeling																								
Crawling																								
BALANCE																								
In sitting																								
In kneeling																								
In standing																								
WEIGHT TRANSFERS																								
Over affected hip in sitting																								
Over affected arm in sitting																								
Over affected leg in standing																								
Over affected arm in standing																								
Over semi-flexed knee in standing																								

Grading: O = NIL   3 = FAIR
1 = MINIMAL   4 = GOOD
2 = POOR   5 = RESTORED TO NORMAL FUNCTION

FIG.80

SIGNATURE OF PHYSIOTHERAPIST _____

Previous Exercise Tolerance ?

Present Exercise Tolerance ?
(eg. cardiac complications)

Is patient's OUTLOOK hopeful ?

Is patient's OUTLOOK hopeless ?

Is VISION normally defective ?

Is HEARING normally defective ?

Cortical integration and sensory interpretation – tactile and postural sensitivity : tested with the eyes covered.

DATE							
Pin - prick							
Joint position							
Light touch							
Two point							
Size and texture							

Fill in : PASSED , FAILED or UNCERTAIN.

Test for HEMIANOPIA : Does the patient ignore visual stimuli on the affected side ?

Test for APRAXIAS : failure to integrate acts into sequence : copy these drawings Neglect of space on either side.

Test for visual AGNOSIA :

DRAW A CLOCK / MAN / HOUSE

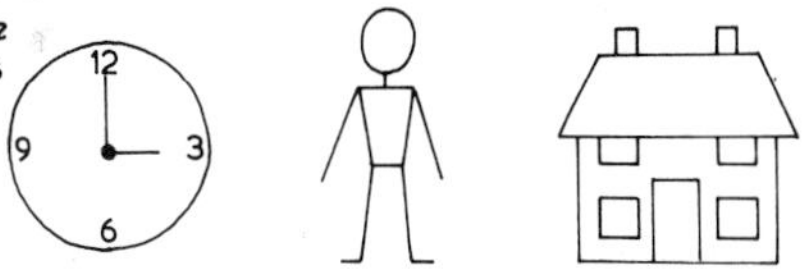

DATE OF TEST	COMMENT

MENTAL CAPACITY : How does the patient respond to simple questions ?

FIG. 81

three may co-exist. 'Stovepipe' rigidity and/or clonus *may* be present (e.g. Corpus Striatum involvement where rolling *must* be re-established if rehabilitation is to make any progress).

3. Evaluation of activities may also be used as a progress report. It is helpful to set out this section of the assessment sheet as a routine progression of physical ability so that no necessary step in rehabilitation is omitted. For example, if the patient fails to establish the degree of active hip control necessary for bridging, why expect him to transfer his weight over his affected hip in kneeling with forearm support? Or, if the patient has not established full kneeling, why expect him to crawl? This means that where grading is concerned, each progression should at least reach a necessary 3 before the next progression is attempted. This does not apply to the activities which are begun at the same time— particularly rolling and bridging.

4. Previous and present exercise tolerance must be taken into account. This means that the physician/physiotherapist relationship must be good with full communication taking place and, where necessary, G.P. and family help is also sought.

5. The state of the patient's outlook ought to be included on the assessment sheet. The patient's outlook must be hopeful. If it is hopeless, the first requirement for successful rehabilitation is missing and the physiotherapist and all who deal with the patient must work towards altering his gloomy outlook. To demonstrate progress (however little) in the early dark days almost always raises morale and the physical method used here gives very early independence (however little) and does not defeat the patient.

6. The importance of knowing the state of the patient's vision and hearing before his stroke makes it necessary to give this point a place on the assessment sheet.

7. Tactile and postural sensitivity must be carefully assessed for what must now be very obvious reasons. For example, it is now fully understood that any loss in proprioceptive sense must be picked up in the very early days and measures taken to step up sensory input so as to make rehabilitation possible. The significance of a brief note 'joint position' must not be overlooked and the importance of this brief note, charted as it is here, can be seen at a glance.

8. Hemianopia and visual agnosia must not be confused. This point has been fairly adequately discussed and the need for charting the results of these tests will be understood.

9. Drawing tests should be carried out on separate clean sheets of paper using a felt-tipped pen. In other words, the three drawings suggested on the assessment sheet are there simply as a visual reminder for the physiotherapist. If she wants her patient to draw a clock she gives him a blank sheet of paper and says: 'I want you to draw a clock face with the numbers on it.' She must stay beside him so that she may watch and assess his performance. If she was testing for apraxic problems she

would draw a two-dimensional house and ask her patient to copy it. Or she might simply draw a two-dimensional diagram, e.g. a box. All drawings to be copied are done in the presence of the patient. A space must be set aside on the assessment sheet for the *date of test* and for the physiotherapist's *comment*. The comment will sum up the drawing tests it might read: 'Neglect of left half of space' or 'Major perceptual disorder' or 'Agnosia and disturbance of body image'. If any of these difficulties are uncovered by the tests it seems fairly obvious that more space is needed for further comment and it will be necessary to add another sheet to the assessment table.

10. Mental capacity might be better if it were headed orientation, simple questions testing memory and awareness of environment. This test will not be suitable for the deaf or aphasic patient. Example of questions asked:

'What is your name?'
'What is your address?'
'What day is it?'
'What month is it?'
'What year is it?'
'What time is it?' The patient is allowed to consult his watch or a clock, or to give the time to the nearest hour.
'What hospital is this?'
'How long have you been here?'
'What is your date of birth?'

Recent memory may be easily and simply tested by the physiotherapist. For example, she may remove the patient's shoes for an exercise session and say to him: 'Look, I am putting your shoes in the cupboard'. Ten minutes later she will ask: 'Where are your shoes?'

Many of the suggested tests are not suitable for the aphasic patient. The definition of *aphasia* is an inability to express thought in words; loss of the faculty of interchanging thought, without any affection of the intellect or will. *Dysphasia* is a disorder of language which may, or may not, include difficulty in comprehension. More usually, comprehension remains intact. *Dysphasia* may give *receptive* or *expressive* or *mixed language disorder*. For this reason it is probably best to note any difficulty in this area at the beginning of the assessment sheet. Any other comment on speech difficulty might be added on the suggested third sheet of the chart.

If not included on the sheet, as it has not been included here, the patient's state of continence or incontinence ought to be recorded. Twenty per cent of old people have trouble with incontinence and this figure will be higher among the elderly stroke patients. It may, for example, be an indication of depression exacerbated by grey surroundings and the social indignity of stroke illness, or it may indicate extensive brain damage that removes social inhibitions, or it may simply be the result of thoughtless prescription of drugs, less awareness of bladder

EVALUATION OF SELF-CARE ACTIVITIES

TRANSFER	AIDED	UNAIDED
From Bed to Chair:		
From Chair to Commode:		
Chair to Standing:		
Chair to Walking:		
Walking to Toilet:		
Dressing:		
Feeding:		
Washing:		
Gait:		
Stairs:		

ANY OTHER RELEVANT COMMENTS:

FIG.82

sensation or loss of tone. With the persistently incontinent, eighty per cent will have brain damage.

Note: A breakdown in communication will be discussed below.

Figure 82 shows the suggested third sheet of the assessment chart. As it would have two sides there would be one and half clear sides for the physiotherapist to add *any other relevant comments.* This seems a reasonable space. As suggested here, this would mean that the physiotherapist's stroke assessment chart would be contained on both sides of two cards which would make for easy handling; assessment and progress would be seen at a glance and the simple layout would be readily understood by all.

The tests suggested are very simple and quick to carry out and, where an area of disability is uncovered, the occupational therapist and speech therapist have much to contribute towards a more detailed and careful assessment. The average physiotherapist might very well miss a high level receptive disability, say, for example, the patient with intact motor function but persistent lack of stability and a lateral lean towards the affected side. Any obscure disability must be identified because the appropriate measures must be taken if the patient is to have any hope of any sort of return to normal living. Suppose, in the case quoted here, with the help of the good physician, occupational therapist, or speech therapist, ideomotor apraxia is diagnosed, the physiotherapist must then decide what she can best do to help the patient. Also, as can happen, suppose the physiotherapist has not got the help of others to pinpoint the difficulty, ought she not to have a fair idea herself of the possible tests she can make to help her to understand her patient's difficulty? I would suggest that where the unfortunate victim demonstrates severe ideomotor apraxia he must at least be given a sporting chance and offered a suitable course of intensive physiotherapy. Again, the aim will be to work on the reflex arc, stimulating reflexes over and over again, attempting to consolidate and stabilise reactions because of the fundamental tendency for nerve cells to repeat an activity. The patient will be taught to work with rolling routines until he establishes rolling to elbow propping, rolling to sitting, rolling to prone lying with forearm support, kneeling with forearm support, full kneeling, crawling and stand kneeling. (It is possible, I quote an actual case.) Balance in these positions must be established and thoroughly stabilised before standing is attempted, and balance in these positions will only be established by intensive methods and very careful positioning to inhibit the dominating reflexes. In the case quoted, the dominating reflexes began to give a build-up of hypertonicity almost immediately after the onset of the stroke. Careful positioning included the need to give the patient constant reminders to use the handclasp position, fingers interlaced, palms touching.

In this instance, careful positioning meant *careful positioning.* For example: (1) Because of ideomotor difficulty the patient had to be *helped* and *reminded* to use the handclasp position all the time in rolling and resting. (2) Also, he had to be reminded over and over again that he must not rest in the supine position. 'Roll onto your side,' was the constant reminder. Or, 'All right, lie on your back if it is comfortable but *not* with your legs out straight.' He eventually learned to position his hands and his legs as routine, automatic actions. A book held between the knees when lying in the crook position was again a very helpful aid and the same position with both knees pointing away from the affected side (i.e. affected hip in internal rotation, or the routine position for resting in supine) was also established with the help of a book.

The patient eventually established full kneeling, crawling, stand kneeling and knee walking unaided. Standing balance proved even more difficult but was facilitated by stepping up sensory input by constant use of a mirror and, where walking proved difficult, it was immediately facilitated by changing the command that was given. With supporting assistance the patient was told: 'Walk with me across the room. Lift your right foot!' He remained glued to the spot. The command was given again, slowly and deliberately. He made a tremendous effort, lifted his affected leg and lost his balance. With continued supporting assistance, the patient was then told: 'Your coffee is over there on the table. Do you want some coffee? Go on then, *go and get your coffee!*' He walked straight across the room with a firm, balanced gait. Using this method his progress was surprisingly satisfactory.

How can we say then, that it is not the physiotherapist's job to assess her patient thoroughly? If she is not capable of thorough assessment she is not qualified to face the more obscure and difficult problems she will inevitably encounter in her work with stroke patients—she won't even recognise them. The assistance and cooperation of a highly qualified occupational therapist and a skilled speech therapist is of enormous help. The more the physiotherapist understands the more she will appreciate and seek out their help. Where relationships are right, each will share enough of her specialised skill to give common understanding. We must be prepared to say: 'I don't know,' and then go out and look for the answer.

Conclusion

Stroke assessment ought to be undertaken with care and understanding so that the physiotherapist may have a complete picture of each patient's area of disability if she is to make a worthwhile and intelligent approach to rehabilitation.

A breakdown in communication

In *The Stroke Patient: Principles of Rehabilitation* I have already dealt quite adequately with this problem from the physiotherapist's point of view. It should, therefore, suffice to repeat little more than the definition and the few points that must be stressed.

1. *Dysphasia* is a *disorder of language* which may include understanding, speaking reading and writing. It is a disorder of the system of communication through the medium of language and leads to an emotional and social breakdown.

2. *Dysarthria* is a *disorder of speech* which includes difficulty in articulation due to neuromuscular defect of lips, tongue, palate and larynx. It is a disorder of expression involving voice, resonance and articulation. There is *no* language loss—therefore, incoding and decoding remain quite normal.

1. *Dysphasia* may be:
(a) Expressive
(b) Receptive
(c) Mixed

(a) *Expressive dysphasia* is an impairment of the output of language and may be referred to as expressive, executive or motor dysphasia. Comprehension remains comparatively intact but the patient can't find words and therefore his output is limited or non-existent. Where the condition is *severe* we find the recurrent utterance. Where the condition is *less severe* we find perseveration. Where the condition is *much less severe* we find social speech is maintained and it may be used to manipulate the conversation so that this level of expressive dysphasia may be missed and the speech therapist may not even be consulted. The speech therapist has ways of inhibiting perseveration, of encouraging fluency and of easing word finding difficulties.

(b) *Receptive dysphasia* is an inability to understand the spoken word adequately. Comprehension is missing and the patient is in the puzzling position of being unable to understand his own language. It may be compared with trying to understand Greek when Greek is an unknown foreign language. The physiotherapist must keep her commands to the bare minimum—very short and very simple—and her commands will be accompanied by manual holds and gentle pressure to facilitate the required response. The speech therapist has ways of inhibiting jargon, of getting the patient to listen to her commands and then of getting him to listen to himself.

(c) *Mixed expressive/receptive dysphasia* simply means that difficulty in comprehension is added to the already difficult problems involved in expressive dysphasia.

The prognosis signs in the dysphasic patient may be *poor* or *good*.
Poor prognosis signs:
(1) Where responses are low to language input
(2) Where there is little or no speech
Good prognosis signs:
(1) Where there is an attempt to use language
(2) Where there is the ability to read
(3) Where there is the ability to write spontaneously.

Assessing speech disability in the stroke patient is a job for the expert and her assessment reports may be used to assist the physiotherapist so that she is better able to approach her part in the rehabilitation plan with greater understanding of the difficulties involved. Not only the physiotherapist, however, but all those who care for the aphasic patient must remember that all of these patients will show the following symptoms:

1. Acute anxiety
2. Exaggeration of previous personality traits
3. Surprising fluctuations in performance
4. Possible 'slow thinking time'.

The necessary allowance must be made for any of these symptoms. Anxiety and tension will inhibit any ability that is present. Again, this means that the physiotherapist and all who care for the patient must remember:

1. To reassure
2. Not to aggravate frustration
3. Not to insist on repetition of single words and phrases
4. Not to isolate
5. Not to lose contact
6. Not to rush the patient—give him time.

The speech therapist has much to offer but she ought to be consulted as soon as possible after the onset of the stroke so that she may establish some form of communication with him at once. Left to himself, the expressive dysphasic patient and the dysarthric patient will both be able to hear and understand their own mistakes and will inhibit any speech they have. This makes the necessity for establishing early communication abundantly clear. Thus, the most important point to remember is that the expressive dysphasic patient *must not* be left to sit helplessly in a corner with complete breakdown in verbal expression and, therefore, with complete breakdown in communication with his family and friends. Time must be taken to educate mankind, at whatever level, wherever he becomes involved in the patient's word finding problem, so that he will understand the patient's communication potential, the reasons for his loss of language, and the best way to help. Family and friends must understand that the patient's comprehension has remained intact and hopeless frustration and loneliness must not be allowed to take over.

Dysphasia may include sensory, visual, auditory and motor defects while *Dysarthria* is a motor defect.

2. *Dysarthria* is less of a problem, but here again cooperation between the two therapists is vital. Articulation and phonation present a clinical picture which demands the attention of both therapists. Again, communication must be maintained.

The clinical picture may show:

(a) Weakness of the soft palate

(b) Tongue deviation with hypertonicity or hypotonicity
(c) Muscle weakness
(d) Drooling.

Speech will be slow, slurred and monotonous. The initial speech sessions give speech encouragement. In the language of the speech therapist, her treatment in this case is to give unremitting voice and articulation practice. Exercises are given for the tongue, the lips, in breathing, in using words and phrases; and then, with the encouragement of the speech therapist and the perseverance of the patient, these exercises are incorporated into speech.

The physiotherapist's part in rehabilitation where there is a breakdown in communication can be vital. Obviously she must establish immediate contact and some form of communication with her patient. An exchange of glances is a beginning. She must, by any and every means she can devise, bridge the gap that threatens to cut him off from his fellow beings in lonely isolation. Family and friends must be asked to help and the patient's former background filled in. His likes and dislikes must be made known. This will include a report on his hobbies, his favourite books, magazines, newspapers, his favourite sport, the football team he supports (if any), the number and names of his children (if any), his favourite radio and television programmes and so on—the list is endless. It is very necessary to have a full picture of his former way of life and a fair estimation of the kind of person he is if a conversation aided by mime and gesture is to be successfully carried out. His physical rehabilitation will go forward along the normal lines and, during treatment sessions, the physiotherapist will have more time with him than any other single member of the caring team who surround him. She will therefore have the greatest opportunity to establish communication. She must help him to compensate for his (hopefully temporary) loss of verbal communication. She must literally take him by the hand and lead him away from what has so suddenly become his very limited and unhappy small private world into the sociable activities that will lead forward towards rehabilitation.

Music therapy has a part to play in treatment of the dysphasic patient. Most of us have come across the singing dysphasic patient who has marked central language disorder with little or no speech and yet is word perfect when singing a former familiar song. This is thought to be because music, as opposed to speech, is interpreted by the opposite (or non-dominant) cerebral hemisphere—or it may be an automatic response.

Every possible means of communication must be used to maintain contact with the patient. So this quite clearly includes, in many cases, the establishment of a non-verbal language in which mime and music have a part to play. Finally, let it be remembered that the infant learns to communicate before he learns to talk. Dysphasia, as I have said, may include sensory, visual, auditory and motor defects. If communication is retained while the physical treatment programme is undertaken and moves forward, speech will improve in the later stages of physical rehabilitation.

In dysarthria where there is a motor defect, obviously the physiotherapist is well qualified to assist in re-education of muscle weakness. A small block of wet ice may be used to good effect to massage affected facial muscles. For ice treatment and for exercise the physiotherapist thinks in terms of muscle direction and she may use her fingers or a wooden spatula to give any desired assistance or resistance. She may work unilaterally or bilaterally and, if necessary, will include eyebrows, eyes, nose and mouth. She may use her fingers or thumbs to depress the eyebrows and then ask her patient to raise them, giving assistance or resistance as necessary. He may be asked to screw up his eyes while she gives resistance to the movement, to sniff against mild resistance given when she closes his nostrils with finger the thumb, and to smile and then to purse his lips with assistance and against resistance. He will be asked to suck against resistance offered by two wooden spatulas which are held inside his mouth with a mild lateral pull to give a wide grin. Finally the tongue is exercised against resistance offered by the wooden spatula and jaw movements are practised. The help of a mirror for facial exercises may be necessary. To assist the exercise of sucking, liquid may be drunk through a straw.

Almost without exception, any work that is done with the patient to assist the speech therapist in re-education of muscle weakness ought to be done in privacy. This type of re-education will embarrass most patients but active cooperation is readily obtained if there is no 'audience'.

Other problems

Mild spasm to severe spasm, mild pain to severe pain, loss of confidence to a feeling of hopeless inadequacy, low morale ranging from disinterested apathy to deep depression and withdrawal into complete isolation are among the problems, or give rise to some of the problems, that may be encountered in stroke treatment. It often does not take many weeks of neglect to produce some, if not all, of these symptoms. We must not delude ourselves into believing that they are simply symptoms of a stroke, and moreover, symptoms that are to be expected after a stroke. They may be—but they are symptoms which can be greatly reduced by competent caring and they are certainly symptoms of neglect which will exacerbate with neglect. I have made a study of results obtained when 'late' treatment has been offered to the neglected stroke patient. Months and even years after onset, if competent physical treatment is offered, morale is immediately raised and relief from the most distressing results of neglect may be had. Perhaps the most tragic case of all is the picture presented by the spastic dysphasic who has sat for years in the corner of a ward in lonely isolation. In other words, the institutional long term case that it is our aim to prevent.

Spasm presents one of the commonest causes of distress which is seen in the tightly fisted hand and painful shoulder. The hand remains useless and inadequately washed with neglected finger-nails digging into the palm. This unhappy state need not continue. If suitable treatment is offered—even at this late date—it is possible to obtain relief and often surprisingly spectacular results. This is where the inflatable pressure splint again has a part to play. With work and patience the tightly fisted hand may be uncurled. Manual work on the fingers to uncover the heel of the hand will allow for sharp tapping on this area to further relax the fingers. A pressure splint is applied, even if it is not possible to move immediately into the full anti-spasm pattern for the arm. In cases of very severe spasm it may only be possible to apply a hand and wrist splint in the beginning sessions of treatment. As soon as possible the full arm splint will be used. The arm is placed as nearly as spasm will allow in the desired position. Treatment ought not to hurt. The splint is inflated orally and left in position for five minutes after which time it is removed and immediately reapplied. It is usually found that this second application is more successful, the first attempt having already produced a degree of relaxation—pressure on the finger-tips, one of the key points of spasm control, having done its work. A third application may be made in one treatment session. When the satisfactory anti-spasm position of the arm is obtained with the shoulder in external rotation, the arm is placed in elevation and the splint is left in position for at least twenty minutes. With the splint in place it is possible to begin passive and assisted shoulder movements, to free the scapula in time and to re-educate controlled movement of the shoulder. When this is achieved arm rehabilitation may begin. In my series of photographic slides showing patient progress I am pleased to have a slide which shows a seventy-six year old lady proudly smoking a cigarette. Smoking might not have been very good for her health but it was the only pleasure she had left. She is holding the cigarette between the extended first and second fingers of her *left hand* and lifting it to her mouth. The important point about the slide is that, prior to pressure splint treatment, she had been sitting for four years with an untreated tightly-fisted spastic *left arm.*

With the full arm pressure splint holding the arm in the complete anti-spasm pattern there is, in the majority of cases, an almost spectacular release of shoulder spasm. Where this does not happen it is usual to find contracture of shoulder muscles and an immobile scapula. If the condition is severe, pain will also be severe. It will not be possible to obtain the full anti-spasm pattern in the arm and extra measures must be taken. Where shoulder pain is persistent and severe, in my experience, treatment by *wet cold* has the greatest effect on:

(a) The relief of pain.
(b) The facilitation of movement.

Treatment by wet cold

The effect of *cold* is of proved therapeutic value. Ice is used in order to be sufficiently cold, cold seeming to have an advantage over the effects of heat.

Heat has a superficial effect, relaxes the patient mentally and physically and produces a feeling of lassitude.

Cold has a much less superficial effect, relaxes the area treated, has a damping effect on localised pain and produces a stimulating effect mentally.

Patients very rarely prefer heat to cold once they have had their cold therapy. It may be said that the physiological effects of heat and cold are extraordinarily alike but the effects of cold go deeper, last longer and are therefore of greater value.

Materials needed for treatment:

1. *Ice:* ice at a temperature of about 37° i.e. *not frozen* but a mixture of ice and water. The ice must be in thin flakes with a large surface area. The source of supply may give a little difficulty but most general hospitals have an ice-making machine to give a source for surgery; at home it may be obtained at the bigger fishmongers; or in any situation it may be made in the ice-making compartment of a fridge. If taken out of a fridge it must be wrapped in a towel and smashed with a hammer. It is important to remember that it must be ice made from pure water only. Some commercial firms add freezing agents which means that the ice is too cold and there is a danger of burns.

2. *Cold water*

3. *Several towels:* the towels ought not to be old and worn. They should be terry towels of good quality.

4. *Two buckets.*

Method: for any application, but in this case for the scapula area of a contracted, painful shoulder. Care should be taken to pinpoint and cover the area where pain is acute.

1. Wet the towels in cold water.

2. Put a folded wet towel in the bottom of a clean bucket and pour flaked ice on top.

3. Place a second towel, wet and neatly folded, on top of the first towel and once again pour flaked ice on top. Repeat the operation adding a third towel, topping with a generous supply of ice.

4. Add a generous 'pour' of cold water and leave to 'cook'. Cooking here means leaving long enough for little flakes of ice to cling all over the surface of the folded towels and this will take 3 to 5 minutes.

5. Remove the top towel, roll it up with the ice inside, wring it out by hand, unroll and place the folded towel over the appropriate area with *the ice next to the skin.*

6. Leave in place for two minutes, or until the ice begins to melt.

7. Repeat the application three times.

Effects of the treatment:

1. *On the circulation:* as soon as the cold is applied to the surface there is a constriction of the surface blood vessels and a decrease in the blood supply with a consequent increase in blood supply to the deeper vessels. Very soon the towel begins to warm up. When the towel is then removed the opposite happens, the surface blood vessels dilate and this is apparent by the developing erythema. All the time the towel is in position the physiotherapist should continue to work the forearm and hand into the anti-spasm pattern. The towel is only kept in place for a short time because it warms up and ceases to be effective.

2. *On nerve endings:* cold slows down the speed of the impulses of pain and, therefore, where it is used there is an immediate reduction of pain. For this reason ice is useful in virtually any painful condition. The result may only be temporary but the temporary period is used to assist the physiotherapist to move the limb passively into the required position without hurting her patient. Also, when pain impulses are slowed down, spasm impulses are also slowed down, spasm being a product of reflex arcs working overtime.

Before the introduction of pressure splints to relieve spasm, ice had a place in stroke rehabilitation for this purpose. Needless to say, the pressure splint does not include the shoulder so there is still a place for ice in this area. Where the patient is very elderly, frail, or with cardiac involvement it can be effective to give no more than an ice massage to the scapula area. This is done by using a *small* block of *wet* ice and giving a deep massage with pressure over the contracted area. I would advocate that in this case the treatment be given under the comfort of a radiant heat lamp and followed immediately by brisk rubbing with a warm, dry towel and deep frictions given using warm hands. If it is still considered unwise to use ice in any form (because of the patient's medical condition) the 'old-fashioned' treatment giving deep frictions followed by a comforting and relaxing massage under a lamp should be given. Physiotherapists in the present day rush probably do not give massage nearly often enough. There are those who consider that the Roman methods of stroke rehabilitation were superior to ours and got better results. The Romans used hot baths, massage, heat and passive exercise. This is a point worth thinking about. Certainly the top present day opinion considers passive movement essential for the basic inhibition of dominant reflexes—or as an important part of rehabilitation where excessive tone must be brought under control.

Subluxation of the shoulder

Many physiotherapists worry unnecessarily about subluxation of the affected shoulder in the stroke patient. The flaccid or hypotonic hanging arm *will* subluxate but this is not a factor to which any undue concern ought to be given. The shoulder joint is, at the best of times, dependent on muscular and ligamentous support to maintain articulation of the head of the humerus with the glenoid cavity of the scapula, the long head of biceps having an important stabilising effect on the joint. Without adequate stabilising support, because of the mechanical position of the scapula with the glenoid cavity, subluxation follows. In the early days after onset of the stroke, *if the patient is correctly handled*—and this includes the maintenance of a free scapula—weight-bearing through a correctly positioned shoulder will replace the mechanical stability of the shoulder joint. Pain has nothing to do with subluxation; pain is associated with strained muscles and ligaments from bad positioning and bad lifting, it is associated with an immobile scapula and with spasm and contractures. Thus, in the late treatment as described above, the physiotherapist is dealing with the effects of neglect and bad handling and she must release the scapula before she can make any sort of beginning to re-educate controlled movement in the arm.

The agony shoulder

The agony shoulder in the stroke patient ought not to occur. With the first sign of shoulder pain shown by any stroke patient in the early days after onset, the physiotherapist ought at once to suspect bad positioning or bad handling somewhere in the hospital team and she ought to be ready to teach those who need help in this field. Where practical, she ought also to instruct the patient himself in taking care of his own positioning. If she explains exactly why it is so necessary to maintain correct positioning and how much his future ability depends on it he is usually more than ready to cooperate. She herself will remember to take extra care with his positioning both during resting and exercising periods. For example, rolling exercise must always be carried out by the patient with his hands clasped, palms touching, both arms reaching forward—and, therefore, with his shoulders protracted and externally rotated. With each roll onto the affected side the arms will be moved up a little more into elevation. It may take some days to reach reasonable painless elevation. It must always be remembered that the aim is to give painless treatment which should be enjoyed. Wherever possible, it is important to *hand over the responsibility of maintaining positioning to the patient himself.* After his treatment session he may be left sitting at the large polished table with both of his arms supported and his hands clasped. Reaching forward as far as possible across the table in this position is another very useful exercise. The patient may be left to do this on his own. The table ought not to be too high; in other words, it ought to be low enough to allow for resting periods with the patient leaning forwards, his forearms placed forwards and parallel so that weight is distributed from protracted and externally rotated shoulders to the forearms. The rubber bath mat on the table-top will be necessary here to give enough stability for resting periods. While he is sitting, the patient will also be taught to maintain a good leg position (as already described) and he should be told that, to a large extent, his progress is in his own hands. Most patients with normal comprehension are more than willing to take up the challenge. If the agony shoulder is allowed to develop it will hold up—or even put an end to—successful rehabilitation, preventing rolling, elbow propping, crawling, standing on the hands and all weight-bearing through the affected shoulder. For reasons of position *a sling should not be used.*

These thoughts on the care of the affected shoulder serve to demonstrate the importance of seeing the entire treatment as a whole from the earliest days and of treating the body as a whole functioning unit. This includes positioning the body not only as separate limbs but as a whole and of exercising one area using correct positions and patterns while the area at rest maintains the correct resting position. It means starting from the earliest days with careful assessment and the carefully planned treatment programme that takes every eventuality into account and so does not run into difficult problems because the cart has been put before the horse. Where shoulder difficulty is encountered in the late stages, as has been shown, it is necessary to go right back to the beginning and start with diligent positioning and work to achieve and maintain a freely mobile scapula. In this case the patient's ultimate recovery has been drastically delayed—if not prevented altogether. How much pain and distress he would have been spared if treatment had been more carefully undertaken in the beginning!

Similarly with the leg, the same dismal picture may be presented when treatment has been delayed, poor, bad or inadequate. Where the neglected stroke patient is found to have developed maximum extensor spasticity in the affected leg some weeks after onset of the stroke, it will be difficult to offer effective rehabilitation. But, until we reach a situation where prevention of developing spasticity is undertaken by all members of the rehabilitation team at all times (from the junior nurse to the superintendent physiotherapist), we are going to come across this difficult and usually quite unnecessary disability. In treatment of the leg, where progress is arrested when it ought to lead forward to a normal gait and useful function, it is quite usual to find there has been a build up of extensor spasticity and any rehabilitation given has not included diligent positioning at all times and weight-bearing through a correctly positioned base. Hence the need to assess tonal pattern at regular intervals during the course of treatment and the need to maintain correct positioning at all times.

Extensor spasticity in the leg

If major extensor spasticity has been allowed to develop in the leg we are faced with a very difficult problem. The patient will walk with an awkward gait making maximum effort to swing the affected leg forward in circumduction and this major effort will increase unwanted muscle tone in the affected arm. He will also weight-bear on the forepart of his foot and not through his heel (or on a badly positioned foot) and this will reinforce unwanted muscle tone in the leg. One of the basic principles of our stroke rehabilitation states that *lower limb activity should* **not** *activate the upper limb.* Even the flaccid upper limb demonstrates withdrawal (or scapula movement into retraction) when maximum effort is made with the lower limb and *this is one thing that must be avoided*. So, if the physiotherapist is faced by a patient with extensor spasm in the lower limb and she is going to make a serious effort to rehabilitate him, *he ought not to walk* until she has reduced the spasticity and brought the dominating reflexes under control. This is possible, but only if she stops the patient from walking—and this does not include weight-bearing—and uses every means in the book to reduce the spasticity. The *techniques used here to reduce spasm* will include and progress through the following stages:

1. *Careful positioning* at all times.
2. *Passive movements* in anti-spasm patterns.
3. *Assisted active movement* where the physiotherapist continues to direct and control the movement, inhibiting dominant reflexes and drift into rotation and.the spasm pattern.
4. *Placing and movement* in normal patterns progressing to movement over more than one joint.
5. Re-education of *the feel of normal movement*.
6. Weight-bearing over a *correctly positioned base*. This must include every detail, such as preventing of knee drift with external rotation of the hip at all times in sitting and weight-bearing through the heel in sitting and standing. Weight-bearing in standing must also include the semi-flexed knee.

Full use will be made of:

1. Comparison of movement with the sound limb.
2. The mirror.
3. Demonstration by the physiotherapist.
4. Recognition of passive movement.
5. Every possible means of breaking down the spasm pattern e.g. foam rubber pads will be placed between widely abducted toes—the foam pads will remain in place for standing (and later for walking).

Note: A footboard for bed rest must never be used. It leads to weight-bearing through the forepart of the foot and reinforces dominant reflexes.

The uncontrolled hip

The uncontrolled hip may also present another very difficult problem if it is found to be present many weeks after the onset of the stroke. It sometimes happens that the physiotherapist acquires a stroke patient for late treatment and she finds on assessment that he has no control of the affected hip. He may not even have obtained the stability and control of movement necessary for bridging. Once again it is a case of going right back to the beginning and working through the whole programme necessary to regain controlled movement of the hip *but*, once again, at this late stage it is not always possible to make up the lost ground and the missed opportunity. Indeed, it is usually quite unrealistic to expect (or even to try to obtain) the satisfactory result that has been missed by lack of early adequate treatment.

The pinned hip

The pinned hip frequently seems to present a problem. A pinned fractured neck of femur, fractured either before or after the onset of the stroke, may produce an unexpected pattern of spasm. Instead of the usual extensor spasm, flexor spasm occurs. Treatment in this case will obviously include the urgent need to inhibit flexor spasm and to prevent the fixed flexion deformities that will develop very quickly if nothing is done to prevent them. Full leg pressure splints are a valuable aid to treatment in these cases. I have come across four in the last two years and they responded to pressure splint treatment. Both orally inflatable splints and those giving intermittent pressure were used. For any degree of success in these cases it is vital not to delay treatment. In all stroke rehabilitation treatment when using full leg splints I take the precaution of rolling the leg into internal rotation.

Interruption of a previous normal married relationship

There is no reason to suppose that after the recovery from a stroke there will be any reduction in a previous normal sex drive, nor should the resumption of the previous married relationship precipitate a second stroke. If, or where, loss of sex drive is experienced, the patient and his/her married partner ought together to seek medical help. Fatigue, loss of confidence and fear of precipitating a second stroke may all be simple contributing factors to this unhappy state, a state which can add the final blow to the patient's feeling of utter inadequacy.

Bowel trouble

Bowel trouble is a fairly usual trouble after stroke. Unfortunately it is frequently misunderstood and misinterpreted. It may present as constipation or diarrhoea *but*, where diarrhoea is a persistent complication, it must always be remembered that this can be (and with stroke patients frequently is) a complication of constipation. It results from a leakage past an impacted faecal mass. Loss of tone, inactivity where the patient formerly led an active life and unsuitable diet to control the consequent bowel failure are all contributory factors. This condition was formerly common among children suffering from poliomyelitis and routine manual evacuation of the bowels was standard procedure. I see no reason to suppose that, as in the patient suffering from poliomyelitis, the patient suffering from a stroke should not be expected to have similar problems. I have myself come across this problem in very many stroke victims and I feel very strongly that it is one aspect of treatment that is often sadly neglected. The physiotherapist ought to be aware of the possibility of bowel disorder and its consequences. The patient suffering from constipation feels out of sorts and thoroughly depressed and the effectiveness of his stroke rehabilitation is considerably reduced, if not halted. I would go so far as to say that in some cases the effectiveness of treatment is so badly obstructed there is a reverse into steady physical deterioration. Constipation is a very common underlying cause of depression.

Experience is the best teacher. The problems the physiotherapist will find she has to face when she undertakes the care of stroke patients will be many and varied. The solutions she may find to solve these problems or to alleviate the distress they may cause, can only be suggested or hinted at in a book of this sort. *A thorough grounding in the principles behind successful rehabilitation* coupled with *wide experience* in the handling of this very specialised type of work must surely be the two essential factors which will lead to satisfactory and worthwhile results. No two stroke patients are exactly the same. No two treatment programmes will be exactly the same down to the last detail. It is impossible to lay down a firm line of action which must be followed in every case *but* it is possible and very necessary to lay down first principles which must be followed with a rigid list of dos and don'ts. It is also necessary to approach the work with an *optimistic outlook* and an expectation of final victory over disability. To approach any stroke patient without optimism and hope is to be doomed to failure before rehabilitation has begun. In most cases it is the physiotherapist who must supply the hopeful outlook that is an essential ingredient in the patient's own approach to recovery if he is to reach the goal of final independence that we have set for him. If the physiotherapist is not capable of helping him to make this approach she is working in the wrong field and she need not expect her patient to obtain satisfactory results. He must have faith in her and the treatment she is offering. Rehabilitation that is founded on sound principles will lead to maximum cooperation and to satisfaction. The results that are obtained when rehabilitation is approached in the way that has been suggested here are thoroughly satisfactory.

Neglect of the necessary principles behind successful rehabilitation, inadequate treatment, delay in starting treatment after the onset of the stroke and failure of any member of hospital staff to cooperate over correct positioning twenty-four hours a day can all lead to sometimes difficult (often indissoluble) problems. We are still frequently faced with any, or all, of these circumstances and the physiotherapist must use tact, ingenuity and skill while she maintains a steady refusal to despair if she is to combat the harm that is often unwittingly done. Spasm, pain, loss of confidence and a feeling of hopeless inadequacy, and low morale ranging from disinterested apathy to deep depression may all be encountered in the stroke patient. If physiotherapists are well grounded in the principles behind stroke rehabilitation, and gain a little of the experience that comes with putting these principles into practice, they will be well fitted to tackle and remove the biggest problem of all—*the ever growing pool of stroke victims waiting for rehabilitation.* As physiotherapists, we must concentrate on the preventive side, that is on the side of care that prevents the stroke victim from becoming the institutional long term case. If we do not go out and meet this challenge, and meet it with the knowledge and understanding necessary to give the worthwhile results that will greatly reduce the number who are at present entering the ranks of the severely disabled, then we must lower our heads in shame and admit that we are not good enough. This may be an appropriate place to state that in my experience calipers, braces, walking aids, etc. all aggravate the patient's difficulties and **I do not use them.**

I have hardly touched on one of the basic necessities of all good stroke rehabilitation. This is the need to educate the relatives. A caring relative can be the most important single factor that will lead a stroke victim back to normality. Where there is a caring relative it is more than a kindness to involve them in the rehabilitation programme—it is a necessity. Wherever possible, relatives should be encouraged to sit in on treatment sessions, they should be taught how they can best help in physical handling and week-end home leave from hospital ought to become a feature of rehabilitation as soon as possible.

Add to this another point I have touched on. It is also most important to hand over diligent positioning and the care of the affected limbs to the patient himself. If he can be taught to understand the significance and the importance of this diligent care he will be only too anxious to cooperate.

There is much that has been left unsaid. There has been no mention for example, of the frontal lobe syndrome with its three outstanding symptoms, failure to learn, failure to suppress, and catastrophic reactions—*but* stroke care is such a vast and fascinating subject, in a book of this length there is much that cannot be said. The purpose of this book is simply to give an account of the sensorimotor approach to rehabilitation as seen through the eyes of a physiotherapist. The neuromuscular system works on a finely balanced facilitory-inhibiting principle which maintains normal muscle tone and gains an effective motor response when sensory input, cerebral integration with motor response and the necessary feedback are all functioning. If one or more of these functions is disturbed, or interrupted, by a stroke which causes a brain lesion—or damage to the cerebral connections—the result will demonstrate in one or more of the following ways:

1. Faulty sensory input
2. Poor cerebral integration
3. Inadequate motor response
4. Faulty feedback.

Conclusion

The sensorimotor approach to stroke rehabilitation as described here is a reasoned and satisfying approach which gives consistently good results. With a breakdown in the finely balanced facilitory-inhibiting principle on which the neuromuscular system depends, the physiotherapist must act as an extended facilitory-inhibiting agent until normal responses are re-established and cortical control regained.

Using the methods described here, this is what she has done. She works to:

1. Inhibit dominant reflexes

Brief Summary Chart of Stroke Rehabilitation

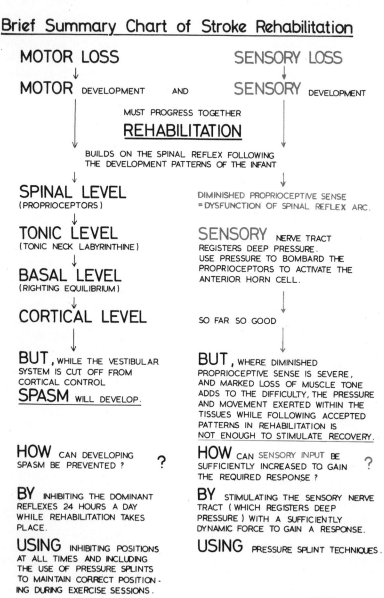

MOTOR LOSS   SENSORY LOSS
↓   ↓

MOTOR DEVELOPMENT   AND   SENSORY DEVELOPMENT

MUST PROGRESS TOGETHER

REHABILITATION

BUILDS ON THE SPINAL REFLEX FOLLOWING
THE DEVELOPMENT PATTERNS OF THE INFANT

SPINAL LEVEL
(PROPRIOCEPTORS)

DIMINISHED PROPRIOCEPTIVE SENSE
= DYSFUNCTION OF SPINAL REFLEX ARC.

TONIC LEVEL
(TONIC NECK LABYRINTHINE)

SENSORY NERVE TRACT
REGISTERS DEEP PRESSURE.
USE PRESSURE TO BOMBARD THE
PROPRIOCEPTORS TO ACTIVATE THE
ANTERIOR HORN CELL.

BASAL LEVEL
(RIGHTING EQUILIBRIUM)

CORTICAL LEVEL

SO FAR SO GOOD

BUT, WHILE THE VESTIBULAR
SYSTEM IS CUT OFF FROM
CORTICAL CONTROL
SPASM WILL DEVELOP.

BUT, WHERE DIMINISHED
PROPRIOCEPTIVE SENSE IS SEVERE,
AND MARKED LOSS OF MUSCLE TONE
ADDS TO THE DIFFICULTY, THE PRESSURE
AND MOVEMENT EXERTED WITHIN THE
TISSUES WHILE FOLLOWING ACCEPTED
PATTERNS IN REHABILITATION IS
NOT ENOUGH TO STIMULATE RECOVERY.

HOW CAN DEVELOPING
SPASM BE PREVENTED ?   ?

HOW CAN SENSORY INPUT BE
SUFFICIENTLY INCREASED TO GAIN   ?
THE REQUIRED RESPONSE ?

BY INHIBITING THE DOMINANT
REFLEXES 24 HOURS A DAY
WHILE REHABILITATION TAKES
PLACE.

BY STIMULATING THE SENSORY NERVE
TRACT (WHICH REGISTERS DEEP
PRESSURE) WITH A SUFFICIENTLY
DYNAMIC FORCE TO GAIN A RESPONSE.

USING INHIBITING POSITIONS
AT ALL TIMES AND INCLUDING
THE USE OF PRESSURE SPLINTS
TO MAINTAIN CORRECT POSITION-
ING DURING EXERCISE SESSIONS.

USING PRESSURE SPLINT TECHNIQUES.

FIG. 83

Summary Chart of Rehabilitation (continued)

USING A CAREFULLY PLANNED PRESSURE SPLINT PROCEDURE, WHICH MUST INCLUDE A SERIES OF PROGRESSIVE EXERCISES, THE SPLINT WORKS AS A MOST EFFECTIVE TREATMENT AID IN STROKE REHABILITATION FOR THE FOLLOWING REASONS:

1. WHEN CORRECTLY APPLIED IT HOLDS THE LIMB IN THE FULL ANTI-SPASM OR RECOVERY PATTERN i.e. IT INHIBITS DOMINANT REFLEXES.

2. IT STEPS UP SENSORY INPUT.

3. IT SUPPLIES THE STABILITY OF SUSTAINED POSTURE THAT IS NECESSARY FOR REHABILITATION.

SUSTAINED PRESSURE IS APPLIED BY USING AN ORALLY INFLATABLE SPLINT — THE WARM, MOIST AIR FROM THE HUMAN LUNGS RENDERS THE SPLINT SOFT AND PLIABLE SO THAT IT MOULDS TO THE SHAPE OF THE LIMB TO GIVE ALL OVER EVEN PRESSURE.

EXERCISE FOR THE ARM MUST INCLUDE WEIGHT-BEARING FROM THE HEEL OF THE HAND THROUGH AN EXTENDED ELBOW TO AN EXTERNALLY ROTATED SHOULDER. THE STABILITY OF SUSTAINED POSTURE OFFERED BY THE SPLINT MAKES THIS EXERCISE POSSIBLE AND EFFECTIVE.

INTERMITTENT PRESSURE IS APPLIED USING A MECHANICAL INTERMITTENT PRESSURE PUMP. WHERE PROPRIOCEPTIVE SENSE IS SEVERELY DIMINISHED AND SENSORY NERVES ACCOMMODATE TO SUSTAINED PRESSURE, MECHANICAL INTERMITTENT PRESSURE MAY BE USED TO GAIN THE REQUIRED RESPONSE.

POSITIONING FOR THE HIP AND SHOULDER IS OF FIRST IMPORTANCE. BOTH MUST BE PROTRACTED WITH THE HIP IN MILD INTERNAL ROTATION, SHOULDER IN EXTERNAL ROTATION.

THE ARM IS MOBILISED INTO EXTERNAL ROTATION.

THE LEG IS MOBILISED INTO INTERNAL ROTATION.

WEIGHT-BEARING THROUGH THE AFFECTED LIMBS IS VITAL TO RECOVERY; THIS MEANS, GRAVITY APPROXIMATION, GRAVITY APPROXIMATION INCREASED BY MANUAL PRESSURE AND FULL WEIGHT-BEARING — ALL TAKING PLACE THROUGH A CORRECTLY POSITIONED BASE —

N.B. WEIGHT-BEARING THROUGH THE HEEL OF THE HAND IS AS IMPORTANT AS WEIGHT-BEARING THROUGH THE HEEL OF THE FOOT.

FIG.84

2. Facilitate reflexes and lost responses
3. Step up sensory input
4. Re-establish lost responses
5. Facilitate effective cortical control and feedback.

The statistician tells us:
1. A stroke is the third commonest cause of admission to hospital
2. There is a very heavy early mortality rate.
3. The survivors have a relatively good prospect,
but
4. There is an ever increasing reservoir of stroke survivors.
5. This represents a tremendous burden on our resources!

Final conclusion

We have not done well enough in the past. *There is much work to be done.* Recovery from a stroke involves a way of life. It is similar to going on to a slimming diet. It is not a way of life that is followed for a few days—or spasmodically—but a way of life that will continue without interruption for many weeks until recovery is complete and it is built round basic positioning. It involves living in the pattern of *recovery* until rehabilitation is complete.

Figures 83 and 84 show at a glance the rehabilitation method for the stroke patient described in this book. These figures are included as an aid to quick revision of the important factors involved and in the hope that they may help towards a full understanding of the method which I have attempted to describe.

Summary of conclusions

1. Voluntary muscles, even when at rest, are always maintained in a state of mild contraction which is called muscle tone and which is more marked in the muscles which hold the body upright against gravity.

2. The factors responsible for the maintenance of normal muscle tone are: the cerebral cortex or other higher cerebral region, the vestibular system and spinal cord, the muscle spindle, and the anterior horn cell.

3. Muscle tone is entirely reflex in character and is directly based on the spinal reflex arc.

4. Where normal muscle tone is missing there can be no normal controlled movement.

5. The missing function that faces all stroke patients is loss of the normal postural reflex mechanism on the affected side; and consequently there will be loss of normal muscle tone with developing spasm, movement loss and usually some degree of sensory loss. *Note:* even where there is a severe degree of hypotonus present, with the passage of time, a developing hypertonus will be found to be present in the anti-gravity muscles.

6. To re-establish normal movement it is necessary to re-establish normal muscle tone. We base our rehabilitation programme on redevel-

opment of the postural reflex mechanism—or, on redevelopment of controlled movement in response to reflex activity.

7. All true stroke rehabilitation must begin at spinal reflex level and work upwards to cortical level. This means beginning at spinal reflex level and working upward to mid-brain responses, using tonic neck reflexes and labyrinthine reflexes, until basal responses are gained, bringing in righting reflexes and equilibrium responses. Basal responses must be established before cortical level can be effective.

8. To follow an effective rehabilitation programme as set out in conclusion 7, the physiotherapist sets out to restore controlled movement following the pattern demonstrated in the motor development of the infant. This development pattern when applied to stroke rehabilitation, is most easily understood and most effective if it is seen and practised as two distinct routines. (a) Rolling to sitting to standing to walking. (b) Rolling to prone to propping to crawling to kneeling to standing to walking.

9. Conclusions 1 and 2 lead to full understanding of conclusion 9. That is the dominating reflexes are modified at cortical level when the postural reflex mechanism is fully established. With the stroke patient this necessary cortical control over muscle tone is lost and abnormal tonic reflex activity gives the typical picture of the spastic hemiplegia. It must not be forgotten that the equally typical picture of the early flaccid hemiplegia will soon develop some degree of spasm (first demonstrated in the finger-tips) and that the extreme degree of flaccidity (or hypotonicity) usually suggests loss of sensation, proprioceptive loss inhibiting the spinal reflex arc.

10. The pattern of spasm bears a direct relationship to the dominating reflexes.

11. The physiotherapist, and all those who handle stroke patients, must act as the inhibiting influence on hypertonic motor neurones until the missing reflex mechanism is re-established and normal inhibiting influences restored. This is done by making sure that the stroke patient is maintained in the anti-spasm (or recovery) pattern twenty-four hours a day and rehabilitation works within this pattern. In other words, correct positioning is used as an inhibiting influence on hyperactive motor neurones (or developing spasm) until inhibition from cortical level is re-established and normal muscle tone restored.

12. All movement of the affected limbs will be passive, assisted and assisted active movements (working through these progressive stages), the operator maintaining the initiative and preventing the release of dominant reflex activity, until static reflexes are integrated into controlled movement.

13. Side-lying positions, which do not increase extensor tone, will be used wherever possible. Therefore, where it is necessary to increase extensor tone in the arm using the supine position and neck extension, the legs will be positioned with extra care. Where it is necessary to leave

the patient in supine lying for any length of time the legs must be positioned with great care and the head will not be supported by pillows to give neck flexion.

14. If early shoulder elevation gives pain it is reasonable to assume that the patient is not being nursed and handled with due care and correct positioning is not being maintained. Also, correct movement patterns may not have been established.

15. To teach the patient to compensate with his sound side is a disservice. For example, to teach him to hook his sound foot under his affected foot to assist its movement is to teach him a habit which will ruin the correct sequence of development of controlled movement and which will later pose very difficult problems.

16. Treatment must be early, intensive and repetitive if worthwhile results are to be obtained.

17. Positioning in the spasm pattern, working into the spasm pattern, allowing drift into the spasm pattern, making excessive demands and encouraging early, willed, voluntary effort will all serve to stimulate unwanted dominant reflex activity and must be discarded from any treatment plan. *This means that the patient will also not be asked to lead an activity with an area of disability until muscle tone is restored to normal.* For example, he should not be allowed to use his hand in any way without forearm support until he can place his arm in space and hold it there.

18. If the spinal reflex arc (which maintains normal muscle tone) is broken by lesion of the motor nerves, the sensory nerves or the reflex centres, muscle tone will be lost. This is because the anterior horn of grey matter in the spinal cord contains vital cells which receive impulses from the proprioceptors along sensory neurones and from the motor area of the cerebral cortex.

19. All movement is a direct response to sensory stimuli from vision, hearing, superficial pressure and deep pressure.

20. If *demand* (or sensory stimulation) from the higher centres of the brain is missing or impaired, it must be stepped up by adding stimuli from the proprioceptors, and, with increased *demand*, a *response* will be gained.

21. With missing or impaired postural, or proprioceptive, sense, sensory input must be stepped up dramatically if there is to be any hope of re-establishing the postural reflex mechanism. Proprioceptors must be bombarded with stimuli until the anterior horn is activated or a response is gained.

22. To stimulate anti-gravity and postural mechanisms we must depend on *weight-bearing*, or *approximation*, and on *deep pressure*— the techniques used to stimulate proprioceptors.

23. Where severe handicap is present because the servo system concerned in anti-gravity and postural mechanisms lacks proprioception, the pressure splint (using both intermittent and sustained pressure) supplies the necessary force to bridge the gap.

24. Where the dominating reflexes are removed from normal inhibiting influences the pressure splint (in this case with sustained pressure and so inflated orally) acts as a most effective inhibiting influence if it is correctly applied.

25. In all cases, weight-bearing through the affected limbs is vital to recovery; this means, gravity approximation, gravity approximation increased by manual pressure and full weight-bearing—all taking place through a correctly positioned base and remembering that weight-bearing through the heel of the hand is as important as weight-bearing through the heel of the foot.

26. The final sequence of distal to proximal movement re-education must be undertaken to reach a satisfactory standard of rehabilitation. Unless the stroke patient is able to *stand on his affected hand* he will not free the primitive flexor grasp and develop controlled hand movements.

27. In the stroke patient, with a breakdown in the finely balanced facilitory-inhibiting principle on which the neuromuscular system depends, the physiotherapist must act as an extended facilitory-inhibiting agent until normal responses are re-established and cortical control regained.

Final summary of conclusions in the use of the pressure splint as an effective aid towards skilled rehabilitation of the affected arm in stroke care. Using a carefully planned *pressure splint* procedure, which must include a series of progressive exercises, the splint works as a most effective treatment aid for the following reasons:

1. It *inhibits dominant reflexes* when it is correctly applied so that it holds the arm in the full anti-spasm or recovery pattern.
2. *Muscle tone* may be influenced by pressure on the finger-tips from the splint, the finger-tips being a key point of control from which the strength and distribution of muscle tone in the rest of the body may be influenced.
3. *Relaxation* of the arm occurs where the Golgi organs are stimulated by contracting muscles pulling on their tendons, prolonged static contraction leading to relaxation. Where the splint is properly applied the necessary prolonged static stretch is made possible. Golgi organs are the specialised sensory receptors, or proprioceptors, in the musculo-tendinous junction and are receptive to stretch. Unlike other proprioceptors, or the stretch receptors of muscle spindles, Golgi organs are known to have an inhibitory effect upon motoneurone pools of their own muscle supply—an autogenic effect. (Autogenic = self-generating).
4. *Sensory input* will be stepped up by the careful and efficient use of the splint.
5. The *stability of sustained posture* that is necessary for effective rehabilitation is supplied by the splint.

For the above five reasons, use of the pressure splint in the re-education of normal function in an arm that has been affected by a stroke makes sound sense. Prolonged stretch of ½ to 1 hour is often found to be most effective.

Exercise for the arm must include weight-bearing from the heel of the hand through an extended elbow to an externally rotated shoulder. The pressure splint makes this possible from an early date.

Intermittent pressure may be given in some cases (using a mechanical intermittent pump) where proprioceptive sense is severely diminished. It makes a useful contribution to treatment where muscle tone is severely lacking but not where there is excessive tone. When used, techniques using sustained pressure should also be included in treatment sessions.

Further reading

The following books are recommended:

Adams, G.F. (1974) *Cerebrovascular Disability in the Ageing Brain.* Edinburgh: Churchill Livingstone.

Bobath, Berta (1970) *Adult Hemiplegia: Evaluation and Treatment.* London: Heinemann.

Cash, Joan (1974) *Neurology for Physiotherapists.* London: Faber & Faber.

Willard, H. S. & Spackmann, C. S. (1963) *Occupational Therapy,* 4th edn. Philadelphia: Lippincott.

The following articles appearing in the periodical *Physiotherapy* are of wide interest:

Vol. 50, No. 1: *Strokes and their Causation* by Helen E. Dimsdale MA MD FRCP.

Vol. 52, No. 10: *Sensory Defects in Hemiplegia* by L. J. Hurwitz MD FRCPE.
Neuroanatomical Aspects and Symptomatology by P. K. Thomas BSc MD MRCP.
Treatment of Hemiplegia complicated by Sensory Defects by G. F. Adams CBE MD FRCP.
Treatment of Acquired Speech and Language Disorders Associated with Hemiplegia by E. Butfield FCST.

Vol. 53, No. 1: *Mat Work* by Helen W. Peterkin MCSP.
Some Aspects of Self-Care by Dorothy Till MCSP.

Vol. 55, No. 4: *Rehabilitation* by A. J. Guymer MCSP.
Neurological Conditions by Ann Brunton MCSP HT & Susan Hunt MCSP DipTP.
The Neuromuscular System and the Re-education of Movement by Helen W. Peterkin MCSP DipTP HT.

Vol. 62, No. 10: *Neurological Mechanisms in Spasticity* by Barry Wyke MD BS
Electromyographic Investigation of Spasticity and Muscle Spasm by J. V. Basmajian MD FACA.
Clinical Features of Spastic States by P. Hudgson MD MRCP FRACP.

Glossary

Active movement. Movement where no attempt is made to assist or resist the action.

Active assisted movement. Movement where the active action is assisted by an outside force.

Agnosia. A perceptual disturbance giving difficulty in recognition.

Agraphia. Inability to express the thoughts in writing.

Alexia. Word blindness: loss of the ability to interpret the significance of the printed or written word, but without loss of visual power.

Aneurysm. Local dilatation of a blood vessel, usually artery, due to local fault in the wall through defect, disease or injury.

Angioma. An innocent tumour formed of blood vessels, usually capillaries.

Anosognosia. Failure to recognise the disability involving the forgotten half of the body: neglect or denial of ownership of the affected limbs.

Aphasia. Inability to express thought in words: loss of the faculty of interchanging thought, without any affection of the intellect or will.

Approximate. To close together with pressure as used when compression is applied through the articulating surfaces of a joint.

Apraxia. A disturbance of visual-spatial relationships, or visual-spatial orientation, which leads to inability to deal effectively with or manipulate objects, or to carry a task through.

Articulation. (as used here) Enunciation of speech.

Assessment. Informal but careful observation leading to a decision on the state of a patient and the line of treatment to be followed.

Astereognosis. Failure to recognise familiar objects by their shape, size and texture when held in the hand with the eyes shut: tactile agnosia.

Body image. The image in an individual's mind of his own body. Distortions of body image occur as a result of affective disorders, parietal lobe tumours or trauma—stroke.

Cognition. Knowing, or awareness, in the widest sense, including sensation, perception etc. Awareness: one of the three aspects of the mind, the others being affection (feeling or emotion), and conation (willing or desiring). They work as a whole but with cognitive disturbance one may dominate.

Corpus striatum. A stalk-like arrangement of grey and white matter at the base of the brain, thought to have a steadying effect on voluntary movement, but no power of initiation of voluntary movement.

Cross facilitation. Working with the sound side of the body across the midline to the affected side to initiate bilateral activity.

Distal. Farthest from the head or source.

Dysarthria. A disorder of speech which includes difficulty in articulation due to motor defect in the muscles of lips, tongue, palate and throat.

Dysgraphia. Difficulty in writing.

Dyslexia. Difficulty in reading.

Dysphasia. A disorder of language which may, or may not, include difficulty in comprehension. More usually, comprehension remains intact.

Equilibrium. Balance: state of even balance: a state in which opposing forces or tendencies neutralise each other.

179

Equilibrium responses. Responses which must include shifts in muscle tone and which make it possible for the body to equilibrate, or to balance or counterpoise, against any altering situation caused by changes of position or environment.

Facilitate. To make easy or easier.

Golgi tendon organs. These are proprioceptors which lie at musculo-tendonous junctions. They are receptive to sustained stretch and are known to have an inhibitory influence on motoneurone pads of their own muscle supply—an autogenic effect.

Hemianopia. Blindness in one half of the visual field of one or both eyes.

Hypertonic. Excessive, or more than normal, tone.

Hypotonic. A lack of, or less than normal, tone.

Ideation. The process concerned with the highest function of awareness, the formation of ideas. It includes thought, intellect and memory.

Ideomotor. Mental energy, in the form of ideas, producing automatic movement of muscles.

Ideopraxist. One who is impelled to carry out an idea.

Infarct. Area of tissue affected when the end artery supplying it is occluded, e.g. in the heart.

Irradiation. Muscle activity which takes place when a strong muscle group acts against resistance to give an overflow of activity (or irradiation) into other parts of the body.

Jargon. Confused talk.

Kinaesthesis. Sense of movement or of muscular effort: perception of movement—adj. kinaesthetic.

Key point of control. Point of the body from which the strength and distribution of muscle tone in the rest of the body may be influenced.

Muscle tone. A state of slight tension of muscle fibres when not in use which enables them to respond more swiftly to a stimulus.

Myocardium. The middle layer of the heart wall.

Neurone. The structural unit of the nervous system comprising fibres (dendrites) which carry impulses to the nerve cell; the nerve itself, and the fibres (axons) which carry impulses from the cell. In the lower motor neurone the cell is in the spinal cord and the axon passes to skeletal muscle. In the upper motor neurone the cell is in the cerebral cortex and the axon passes down the spinal cord to arborise with a lower motor neurone.

Paraphasia. A form of aphasia in which one word is substituted for another.

Parietal lobe. The lobe of the brain which contains the sensory area.

Perception. Act or power of perceiving: discernment: apprehension of any modification of consciousness: the combining of sensations into a recognition of an object.

Perseveration. Meaningless repetition of an utterance (or an action as in drawing): tendency to experience difficulty in leaving one thought for another.

Phonation. Production of vocal sound.

Poly- in composition, many.

Positioning. Placing in the optimum position to allow for, and promote, recovery.

Primitive movement. Movement which is entirely reflex in character, fundamental, belonging to the beginning.

Prognosis. Forecasting, or forecast, especially of the course of a disease.

Proprioceptor. A sensory nerve-ending receptive of sensory stimuli.

Proprioceptive (adj.), pertaining to, or made active by, stimuli arising from movement in the tissues.

Proprioceptive sense. The sense of muscular position, or of muscle and joint position.

P.N.F. Proprioceptive Neuromuscular Facilitation. Methods used to facilitate a response from the neuromuscular mechanism through stimulation of the proprioceptors.

Protract. To draw forward, or lengthen.

Proximal. Nearest to the head or source.

Recovery pattern. The pattern of movement which inhibits dominating reflexes in the stroke patient to allow for, and promote, recovery. This must also include the resting position, which is the position in which the body is placed to allow for optimum recovery while at rest.

Rehabilitation. Obtaining the maximum degree of physical and psychological independence after disability by means of a carefully planned physical programme which must be presented to the patient with cheerful optimism, an optimistic approach being a necessary part of successful rehabilitation.

Resistance. Opposition.

Resisted movement. Movement where resistance is given to gain a greater response, or to strengthen the action.

Retract. To draw back or shorten.

Servo mechanism. A mechanism serving automatically to control the working of another mechanism.

Spasm. A violent involuntary muscular contraction; a state of continuous muscular contraction as opposed to intermittent contraction.

Spatial orientation. Awareness of body position in relation to space.

Stereognosis. The recognition of familiar objects by their shape, size and texture when held in the hand with the eyes shut.

Stimulus. An action, influence, or agency that produces a response in a living organism.

Synapse. The point of communication between two adjacent neurones.

Synergists. Muscles which contract and relax in conjunction with prime movers crossing more than one point. N.B. The synergic pattern of tonic contraction, therefore, results from hypertonic, or excessive, muscle tone leading to muscle contraction which follows the pattern of the synergists.

Vestibular nuclei. These are four in number, superior, lateral, medial and inferior vestibular nuclei which can effect *changes in muscle tone.* In particular it seems likely that connections with the cerebellum are concerned with the postural control of muscle tone. The pathway for transmission of impulses to the cerebral cortex is not clear, but it is thought that connections pass in the posterior thalamus to the temporal lobe. Efferent fibres from the nuclei pass through the length of the mid-brain, hind-brain and spinal medulla and are distributed to both sides.

Vestibular system. The vestibular system is closely concerned in the *postural control of muscle tone in relation to gravitational forces* acting on the maculae of the utricle and saccule, and similar reactions to movement (e.g. maintenance of balance) mediated through the reticular formation—Reference: *Cunningham's Anatomy.*

Appendix—List of useful addresses

Arjo Pilot
  Manufactured in Sweden. Arjo AB, Eslöv, Sweden.
  Arjo U.K. office: 4 Astor Close, Winnesl, Wokingham, Berkshire, RG 11 5JZ.
Calthena Adjustable Plinth
  Supplied by: R. Kincaid & Co., 646 Argyll Street, Glasgow.
Gutter Extension Arm-Rest
  Manufactured in Scotland. Supplied by: J. Buchanan, 52 Dublin Street, Edinburgh.
Polyform (low temperature plastic)
  Made by Rolyan. For further information contact: Rolyan, P.O. Box 555, Menomonee Falls, Winsconsin 53051.
  U.K. Agent: Martin Creasey & Co., 106 Marlborough Avenue, Hull, HU5 3JT.
Pressure Splints
  Urias: Orally Inflatable Air Splints (for sustained pressure)
  Made in Denmark. Marketed by Searle Medical Vallensbaekwej, DK-2600 Glostrup.
  U.K. Office: Searle Medical, P.O. Box 11, Coronation Road, High Wycombe, Bucks. HP12 3TD Or may be obtained from: Whitefield Medical Ltd., 10 Ardmillan Place, Edinburgh, EH11 2JR.

  Jobst: Jet-Air Orally Inflatable Splints (for sustained pressure)
  Made by Jobst: Jobst, P.O. Box 653, Toledo, Ohio 43694
  Marketed in U.K. by Jobst Service Centre, Jobst United Kingdom Ltd., 17 Wigmore Street, London.

  Flowtron-Aire Ltd: Intermittent Pressure Pump and Sleeves.
  Flowtron-Aire Ltd., 5a Lye Trading Estate, 137/141 Old Bedford Road, Luton, Beds.

Selectagrip Cutlery
  From Nottingham Handcraft Co., Melton Road, West Bridgford, Nottingham, NG2 6HD.

Therapeutic Putty
  I have not been able to find a firm that can supply Theraplast. Carter's Therapeutic Putty has proved readily obtainable and equally good.
  Supplied by: Carters, Alfred Street, Westbury, Wilts.

Index